How to
RENEW
YOU

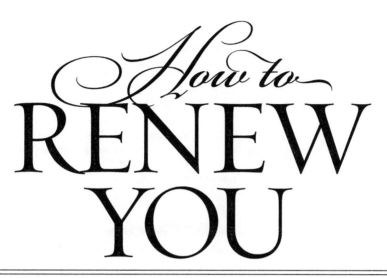

How to RENEW YOU

The Complete Primer on Age Reversal

MAUREEN KENNEDY SALAMAN

MKS, Inc.

How to Renew You
By Maureen Kennedy Salaman

Copyright © 2003
by Maureen Kennedy Salaman

ISBN: 0-913087-17-3 Trade paper
ISBN: 0-913087-22-1 Hardcover

First Edition

Published by:
MKS, Inc.
1259 El Camino Real, Suite 1500
Menlo Park, California 94025

www.mksalaman.com

(650) 854-3922 telephone

(650) 854-5779 facsimile

Distributed by:
Maximum Living, Inc.
20071 Soulsbyville Road
Soulsbyville, California 95372-9748

www.maximizeyourlife.com

(209) 536-9300 telephone

(800) 445-4325 toll-free

(209) 536-9375 facsimile

Interior and cover design by:
Koechel Peterson & Associates, Inc., Minneapolis, MN

Printed in the United States of America

IMPORTANT NOTICE

This book is neither a medical guide nor a manual for self-treatment. It is instead
intended as a reference work only. The information in this book is meant to help you
make informed choices about your health, but is not intended as a substitute for any
treatment that may be prescribed or recommended by your doctor or health care practitioner. If you should suspect that you suffer from a medical condition or problem, you
should seek competent medical care without delay.

ACKNOWLEDGMENTS

My acknowledgments start with special thanks to my staff for their tireless efforts and dedication. They help lighten my load.

To my inimitable friend and researcher Julia Bauer—the sagacity of your work lights my path and brightens the lives of so many. My thanks also goes out to Shirley Osward for your years of help, support, and devotion.

To the officers, board members, staff, and membership of the National Health Federation: I have served them with passion and dedication for over two decades and for the last 18 years as their President. May God continue to make them brave and keep them true.

To my brother Lieutenant Colonel Thomas C. Gillespie, U.S. Marine Corps, a man of integrity, honor, and brilliance who understands there are worse things than death—there is dishonor, lack of loyalty to your country, your family, and the ideals you hold dear.

To Jackie, my sister-in-law, who must be the world's greatest mother. Her patience, fortitude, and self-sacrifice are examples to all who know her.

To Alexandra and Christopher who give me hope for tomorrow and hope for America in tomorrow.

To my son Sean, who started me on my search for truth, and his beautiful angel Melissa, whom I love like a daughter.

To Nancy Hamon, a woman of remarkable spirit and delicious humor. When I grow up, I want to be just like her.

My friend Sally Jordan's scalpel-sharp wit lifts the clouds of the darkest day. Her discerning grace and elegance epitomizes the American spirit with her creative initiative and enterprise. She is constant and steadfast and loyal, brilliant and beautiful, elegant and giving, thought-filled for others. No finer or truer soul ever graced this earth. Her riveting brilliance and shining literary prose make it more than a privilege to call her my friend. I am rarely happier than when I am in her loving presence.

To Katherine Marcus and her husband, Tom. The forthright Katherine and I share our love of God and Country with equal passion. I find it such confirmation that His hand must have forged us from the same mold. No finer character, no fuller heart was ever forged by God.

To my friend, French Normandy native Maurice Renaud. His magnificent character has led him to continue his family's dedication by solidifying the 82nd Airborne Division. These brave heroes sacrificed their lives to free Sainte Mere Eglise from the boot of tyranny while his father was mayor, therefore winning the decisive battle of WWII and giving the Americas and Europe 50 years of peace, prosperity, and freedom. He dedicates himself to keeping their sacrifices alive in memory and strengthening their bond.

Maurice is brave and bold, kind and wise, fine and true. He is less of a wisher and more a doer—more willing to give than get. Broad and big, he helps others to live. May we all as Americans pray and plea, "Lord, may more of his character be in me."

Scott Tips, Esq., who is that one in 10,000 who has stood with me like a brother, and his wife, Karen.

If I were on a ship in the middle of a storm, I would want the dedicated and hard workers at LeSea Broadcasting Television Network to be my crew. Peter Sumrall, President of LeSea and its driving force, would be my distinguished captain. Peter is a visionary, a man of absolute integrity. Brilliant and forthright, he dedicates himself completely to LeSea Broadcasting Television Network, while raising millions of dollars to support "Feed the Hungry." He steadfastly carries the burdens and responsibilities for LeSea with faith, courage, brilliance, and humor.

LeSea's crew are my family. They work hard, diligently, and brilliantly. Andy Greathouse is our creative cameraman. He makes me look good no matter how I feel. Producer Chuck Huffman is an ingenious genius. No matter where in the world we are shooting, we say, "OK, Chuck, how are you going to outdo yourself on this one?" He always does. The others, as well, I would trust with my life: Doug Bullard, the lighting man; Krista Tepe, on-air commercial; and Craig Wallin, on-air host. The humor we share makes every project stimulating and fun. I am most blessed to work with people I enjoy and care about so deeply.

I learned to be a true friend, not by reading good books, but by experiencing the most trustworthy confidantes and loyal friends the world has ever birthed. They are more than friends; they are my soul mates and support system. The greatest gift God gives is loving friends. In this I am the wealthiest of people. My true wealth is manifest in the following people.

My friends, who bless my life so richly, are: Julia "Cori" Haskett-Abbruszzese and Stefan Abbruszzese, Michele Alioto, an angel who walks on earth and her husband, Joe, Heide Van Doren Betz, Iran and Howard Billman, Norma Bixler, Freda and Claud Bowers and Family, Linda Kurtzig

Breitstone, Barbara Brookins-Schneider and Jim Schneider, Helen Gurley Brown, Ellie and Theodore Brown, Linda Cannon, Dr. Richard Casdorph, Toni Casey, Carolyn Chandler, Mike Colbert, Donna Francis and Don Prospero Colonna (Princess and Prince of Stelighiano), Angela Coppola, Yolande Desjardin, Harry and Margot Dewildt, Donna Douglas, Samantha Duval-Chandler, Oleen Eagle, Dehlia Erhlich, Bella Farrow, Thomas Foran, Pastor Kenny and Shirley Foreman, Alisa and Kenny Foreman, Jr, Dawn and Kurt Foreman, Brigitta Forssius, Charlie Fox, Dr. Michael and Inga Gerber, Gail and Dr. Harvey Glasser, Joel Goodrich, Kathryn Grayson, Fred Haeberlein, Nancy Hamon, Ron Hembree, Fred Hirth, William Holloway, Ana Luz Holloway, René Horsch, Nancy and Jack Horton, Wendy and Frank Jordan, Evelyn Kean, Betty Kimball, Dr. Alan Konce, Dr. Hans Kugler, Mathilda and Dr. Richard Kunin, Nick Lampros and Family, David Lassman, Margaret Lawrence, Howard and Gretchen Leach, George Mateljan, Dave McAllister, Ruth and Merl McAnich, Michael and Hershey McKenna, R.J. Merck, Nolan Miller, Billie and Dr. Ralph Miranda, Scotty Morris, Cher and Chris Mullen, Carol Ann and Martin Newman, David Pace, Michael Piombo, Silvia and Joe Pravenzia, Bob Pritikin, Jimmy Reeves, Burt Reynolds, Mary and Dr. Henry Ritter, Jerry Roberts and Family, Dr. Rodrigo Rodriguez, Rob Rosenberg, Janet and Michael Savage, Cynthia Schreuder, Patricia Sinclair, Becky and Tom Smith, Stephanie and Rob Soufla, Betsy Spohn, James Strock, Phyllis and Dr. Murray Susser, Jeanne Taylor, Elizabeth Theriot, JoAnn and Jimmy Thompson, Dr. William and Jo Toy, Princess Paul of Romania (Lia Triff), Dr. John Trowbridge, Alan and Barbara Virchow, Angela Von Hohenzollern, Katherine Wells-Debs, and Mark Zunino.

CONTENTS

BIOGRAPHY

MAUREEN KENNEDY SALAMAN'S life-enhancing messages encompass her unique combination of talents and capabilities that have impacted the billions of readers of her books, articles, tapes, television viewers, and live audiences around the world. Maureen's accomplishments could literally fill volumes. For over a quarter of a century, she has dedicated herself to one goal:

"Empowering people with the right information necessary to maximize their personal health and well-being."

Maureen is an award winning author of six books—*Nutrition: The Cancer Answer, Nutrition: The Cancer Answer II, The Diet Bible, Foods That Heal, The Light at the End of the Refrigerator — The Foods That Heal Companion Cookbook,* and, her monumental encyclopedia, *All Your Health Questions Answered Naturally.* Her cutting edge, best-selling books have sold millions throughout the world to people seeking nutritional answers to health problems. She is published regularly in newspapers and magazines throughout North America and supplies a weekly column for one of the largest online newspaper networks on the Internet.

Maureen is not only an award-winning writer, but a concise and compelling speaker of extraordinary ability. In constant demand, she shares her wisdom, wit, and insight as a media guest for television and radio.

She delivers her health and motivational messages to approximately 20 million people monthly throughout the U.S., via live interactive television as well as the world via satellite. She has shared the wit, wisdom, and insight of her health and motivational messages at over one thousand engagements in the past two decades and in over 300 cities in America and around the world.

Hugely sought after by the public and media, Maureen has toured Australia, Canada, Europe, Japan, the Orient, and the continent of Africa speaking to audiences on natural healing and its beneficial lifestyle. She has hosted the Angel Award winning television program *Accent on Health* and an informational talk show *The Informed Viewer*, as well as thousands of live and pre-recorded television and radio broadcasts. Her award-winning television shows have run continuously since 1983.

Maureen holds a Ph.D. and was valedictorian of her class at the International University of Nutrition Education of Huntington Beach, California. She has a Ph.D. in science from Oral Roberts University, in Tulsa, Oklahoma, a degree in Theology from the California School of Theology, Orange County, California, and a Ph.D. from the British Guild of Drugless Practitioners, Edinborough, Scotland. Maureen continues her educational growth by working with leading institution research teams throughout the world.

Maureen's world-wide research and writing in the field began 37 years ago with an attempt to save her beloved friend Helen Sweet, who was dying of cancer. As a highly respected and regarded author in the field of health and nutrition, she is in touch with the wellness challenges confronting people of all ages and every day is able to share, through her books, television shows, newsletters, radio programs, research, writing, and experiences, what works, what doesn't work, and why.

Maureen is listed in *Who's Who of Editors and Authors*, *Who's Who of America*, *Who's Who of American Women*, and *Who's Who of the West*. She was awarded the "Right Stuff" award from the distinguished Life Center of Houston, Texas. Serving for 18 years, Maureen is the longest elected president of the National Health Federation, the oldest and largest health freedom organization in the world.

FOREWORD

by Murray Susser, M.D.

I HAVE KNOWN MAUREEN KENNEDY SALAMAN AND HER WORK FOR OVER TWENTY YEARS. Her work is beautiful and brilliant, and never has writing been more of an embodiment of the writer than with Maureen. Her latest work reaches even beyond her tradition of packing volumes of valuable and entertaining information into a framework of literary, scientific writing.

Maureen creates an "oxymoron" of style by blending scientific nutritional scholarship into a highly literate tour de force. I have always thought that we learn more from teachers who can frolic with the subject rather than stultify us with pedantry.

This book frolics with us from the present marvels of the arts and sciences of longevity to the futuristic possibilities that entice us into being grateful to dance this computerized yellow brick road to the Land of Awesome—the land of long and healthy lives.

Here we can cover the gamut of the various aspects of longevity. Maureen skillfully guides us on a tour of the mind, the spirit, and the bodily chemistry that offers us the best of all possible bodies to house the life force. Merely staying alive does not define longevity in the view of this book. Nor have I ever known anyone who wants to live out their dotage disabled or unconscious (although the actor Christopher Reeve bravely demonstrates how life can be rich, even as a quadriplegic). Nor will we accept a healthy body with no purpose to pursue. Living long and strong can give us longevity. But how empty without goals and purpose to define our life beyond mere existence. We want to be happy and productive. To accomplish this, we must have philosophy and consciousness. Maureen masterfully takes our spirit through our social world into the future that defines the path to these solutions.

Thus, we see in this book the gleaming synthesis of the essential elements of longevity. This is simply what I want out of a book on living long. I want information on how to do what I can for myself and beyond that, where I can find help for what I cannot do for myself. Maureen easily gives me that approach in this book. I can use the information in this book to increase my life quality and length beyond the ordinary. Thus, the book gives me the tools to have an extraordinary life. Now, it is true that I live and use many of these techniques in my own practice, both for my patients and myself. Yet, I learn much from this book. I have lived and studied this philosophy for about thirty years, but I can use this book as a reference source. I can refresh what I already know, and learn newly what I have not yet encountered. What more can any seeker of truth ask from life?

I shall close the circle by saying that Maureen walks her talk. She lives as she preaches. She is beautiful, youthful, energetic, strong, athletic, spiritual, loyal, and phenomenally productive. I could have gone on with the adjectives, but it may seem unbelievable. She writes in the rich literary style of a sophisticated novelist while she teaches us simply like a favorite teacher from high school. This is no small accomplishment.

I suggest that everyone I have ever known could benefit from this book. And I have known, personally, many of the great leaders in the field of longevity and nutrition. I have known Carlton Fredericks, Linus Pauling, Adelle Davis, and many more such luminaries. I believe that Maureen Kennedy Salaman continues their great legacies. I have learned from all of them and many more. I feel privileged to be able to be here at the onset of another milestone in this great tradition.

How to
RENEW YOU

1

*" Go confidently
in the direction of your dreams.
Live the life
you have imagined."*

HENRY DAVID THOREAU

CHAPTER ONE

THE NEW PHILOSOPHY OF AGING

The Benefits of a Youthful Attitude and Healthy Habits

he journey to living younger longer is a continuous one. It started when you chose to read this book. Your choices, just like the food you eat, are what make you the person you are, and the person you want to be. Every day you can choose to be whatever you want. You don't fail until you give up, so don't give up. If it takes six months to attain your desires, so be it. If it takes six years. . .never give up.

RATHER THAN BECOME VICTIMS OF "THE MYS-TIQUE OF AGING"—the idea that aging equals frailty—each of us has the ability to attain the full human potential of the new years of life beyond our youth—"the third age," as the French call it.

Researchers have much to support the concept of "productive aging." New types of intelligence more than make up for rote memory losses. The capacity for friendship and making new friends remains unchanged by time. People can have an active, fulfilled love life well into their 80s and beyond.

In studies of the lives of men and women (now in their 70s) who were followed since their teens, researchers found the biggest predictor of happiness—more than money, marriage, or health—was spending time doing the things that give them the greatest sense of meaning and allow them to most fully express who or what they consider themselves to be.

RETAINING THE VIGOR OF YOUTH

Human beings are designed to retain the traits normally associated with childhood throughout our adult lives, a process known as neoteny. These traits include curiosity, imagination, playfulness, open-mindedness, willingness to experiment, flexibility, humor, energy, eagerness to learn, and perhaps the most pervasive and most valuable of all, the need to love.

What we must guard against is a hardening of the mind—I call it arteriosclerosis of the attitude—that discourages us from encountering anything new or unfamiliar. In the same way we need to cleanse our arteries of cholesterol accumulations, we need to rid ourselves of the crusty behavior we associate with adulthood and open our hearts and minds, as we did as children, to the world around us. I strive to learn something new and make a new friend every day of my life.

Imagine what life could be like if it were not only disease-free, but also complete with a wellspring of ever-present energy in your waking hours. It would allow us to wrestle challenges into shape and master them with greater satisfaction than previously experienced. Imagine waking up each day ready and eager to face the world and the challenges that lie ahead. The choice is yours, and it is literally a choice between life and death. Throughout this book I will endow you with knowledge *you* need to make that choice. You will have to take it from there and remember that only *you* have the power to make it happen.

In the pages that follow, you will find answers to your concerns about getting older; including, but not limited to, (1) the philosophies others have incorporated into their own lives that will show you how to develop the heart, confidence, and inspiration to live an active, fulfilled, and better life; (2) nutritional solutions to the ailments, syndromes, and diseases that typically shorten your life and limit your choices; (3) tips and techniques to improve what you see in the mirror; and (4) how your relationships with others guide, restore, and heal you, and can add vibrant decades to your life-span.

The desire to live a long life, while important, is not enough. What is required is nothing less than the willingness to change your perception of aging.

In the 20th Century alone, we added 25 more years of life expectancy, the equivalent of half a lifetime at the turn of the last century. Just think how much we can, and will add in the next 50 years.

The desire to live a long life, while important, is not enough. What is required is nothing less than the willingness to change your perception of aging; make the appropriate lifestyle changes, and affirmatively change your life.

HOW LONG CAN WE EXPECT TO LIVE?

As a result of superior sanitation—flushing toilets, running water, and hygiene standards—many of the major causes of death in youth and middle age have been eliminated. Today we can look forward to an average life expectancy of 75 years for men and 80.9 years for women. Six out of ten people with whom you attended high school will die of heart disease. Heart disease is easily our number one killer. Curing cardiovascular disease would practically close the mortality gender gap and boost average life expectancy by about 14 years. According to the California Health Department, wiping out but one major risk factor, arteriosclerosis, would increase the life expectancy of California women to 100 years.

Numbers are helpful; however, we are individuals, not statistics. By making the right choices, we can vastly improve our prospects for a long, vigorous, and healthy life and live well beyond the *average* life expectancy. The Biblical promise in Job 5:26 was that Job would "come to thy grave in a full age." For Job, that "full age" was 120. Genesis 6:3 states that "man's days shall be 120 years." The Biblical character Methuselah lived for 900 years.

Noted aging researcher Leonard Hayflick, Ph.D., estimates our *potential* life-span to be approximately 115. Jeanne Calment of Arles, France, surpassed that mark by seven years. While no one looks forward to 600 years of playing shuffleboard, the truth is most people who *live longer* also live better. Calment rode a bicycle until she was 100, and that year she walked all over Arles to thank those who had congratulated her on turning 100.

Medical research is beginning to realize the Biblical edict. The discovery and understanding of telomeres, the tails of DNA, are helping scientists fulfill God's 120-year promise. Virtually all types of body cells, except reproductive cells, contain this aging clock. It consists of a strand of DNA on the end of all chromosomes. These ends are called telomeres, and every time a cell divides some of this tail is used up. Thus, we eventually run out the aging clock until the cells in our bodies stop dividing. This cellular aging phenomenon is known as the "Hayflick Limit."

The maximum life-span of a species is determined mainly by the number of its cell divisions, measured by the number of subunits on a telomere. The maximum number of subunits that human telomeres have is 60, corresponding to a potential maximum of 60 cell divisions, and translating into a maximum life-span of *120 years*! Science has now proven the Biblical promise that we have a potential life-span of 120 years and beyond.

With respect to our "life-span," science is finally catching up with what was stated in the Bible more than 500 years ago. Furthermore, the potential for additional merging between the Scriptures and science grows almost daily. Scientists have now learned how to unlock the secrets of the telomeres. Through a process by which human stem cells are replicated (thereby restoring the length of the telomere), it may soon be possible to regrow a damaged heart and regenerate the skin. Some say science, as it has already proven with some farm animals, will one day be able to replicate the entire human body. Keep in mind, also, that replicating a cell means if there is any error in that DNA, it will be multiplied and magnified, thus passing on the magnified abnormality. This is where the line will be drawn. You may be able to replicate and/or reproduce each and every body part, but no one can replicate the spirit and soul. Those are bestowed, by God, upon each of us, individually, and no scientist, regardless of his or her brilliance, possesses that capability. Notwithstanding the very real ethical issues associated with this process, this new technology shows promise not only in its potential for lengthening life but also for its potential use in curing age-related disorders.

YOUR BILLION DOLLAR MACHINE

Dr. Edward Teller, the great atomic scientist known as the Father of the Hydrogen Bomb, said that if we could harness the electrons that spin around in the atoms that make up the human body, our bodies could fuel a large industrial nation for more than a week. Think about it. The electrons in our body have the potential to exert eleven million kilowatt hours per pound!

Electrons spark the activity of the heart, which is what electrocardiograms measure. And what sparks the electrons?

Minerals—nutrients essential to our bodies. Never underestimate the value of nutrition in health and longevity. Nutrition is the oil that lubes and the gasoline that fuels your engine.

Imagine for a moment that you have an automobile that can repair itself. You back out of a parking lot and put a dent in your fender the size of a canned ham and in a few weeks the dent has closed itself up, the paint is refinished, and the repair is so perfect you can't find a trace of the accident. Would you be interested in owning such a car?

There exists such a self-repairing machine, and it is the most magnificent machine ever created, and I do mean *created*—a machine that is, in biblical terms, "wonderfully and fearfully made."

No matter how old you are or what condition you are in, you can and must change your life today, and if you do, all your tomorrows will be different.

No doubt you've already guessed it—your body. The very same body that for years you may have abused, reused, fueled improperly, and taken for granted. And yet in spite of the damage it may have sustained, in the time it takes to read this chapter, over seven billion cells will renew, rebuild, and refurbish themselves. Consider this. Each cell of the body has a brain that enables it to heal, refurbish, and upgrade itself.

You didn't need a doctor to grow up. It grew and healed itself. The body's innate intelligence is infinite. Given the chance, and without interference from free radicals, our bodies can, will, and do heal themselves.

More than 2,000 years ago, Hippocrates, the father of modern medicine, was aware of the body's healing powers. He observed that people who had inoperable cancer outlived those who had their tumors surgically removed. What was his prescription? Simply put, it was, "Let medicine be your food and let food be your medicine."

ESCAPING THE NURSING HOME

Over the past twenty years, a number of studies have shown that the people who treat the elderly, make decisions regarding the elderly, and even those who research the elderly hold negative perceptions regarding the aged, viewing them as childlike and dependent, and nursing homes as places where we send people to die. In one study, most of the surveyed decision-makers believed that five times as many people over 65 were institutionalized than was actually the case. The truth is that less than five percent of the over-65 population group are in nursing homes. Many are choosing to forego retirement in favor of fulfilling work, with companies eager to hire them.

One such company is Bonne Bell, a $100-million family owned cosmetics firm based in a working-class neighborhood outside Cleveland. Jess Bell, the 76-year-old son of the company's founder, oversees a seniors-only production department where the average age of the 86 assembly workers is 70 and the oldest is 90. It was not a grand social experiment, but a practical business move. The company needed workers, and seniors were available. Retirees account for 20 percent of Bonne Bell's work force of 500. Since the department was mobilized, Bonne Bell has seen a profit increase of more than $1 million, effectively silencing skeptics.

HEALTH SPAN, NOT LIFE-SPAN

What really matters is how long we stay healthy, not how long we live. The new focus is not on life-span, but on health span. Disease, not age, is the villain. Disease is the enemy we need to defeat.

The beautiful part is, it is *never* too late to start. No matter how old you are, what condition you are in, how poor your lifestyle habits have been, you *can and must* change your life today and, if you do, all your tomorrows will be different.

Fred Astaire said, "Aging is like everything else—if you are to do it well, you must start young."

"People practice to get old," said the late, great George Burns. "The minute they get to be 65 or 70, they sit down slow, they get into a car with trouble. They start taking small steps."

When somebody took leave by telling 100-year-old Jeanne Calment, "Until next year, perhaps," she retorted, "I don't see why not! You don't look so bad to me."

WHAT A DIFFERENCE OUR CHOICES MAKE

Long-term studies by experts in top research institutions around the world confirm that men and women who practice good health habits live longer and do better physically than those who don't.

In Holland, ice skaters had a 24 percent lower rate of death from all causes compared to the general male population. In one insurance study, 2,000 people who practiced stress-reduction techniques had 87 percent less heart disease, 55 percent fewer malignant tumors, and 87 percent less nervous disorders than the general population. In Norway (over the course of a 16-year study period) physically fit middle-aged men had half the death rate of sedentary men. A decade-long California study of more than 11,000 men and women found that vitamin C in amounts equivalent to two oranges, plus 150 milligrams of supplemental vitamin C, lowered the risk of death from heart disease by 42 percent in men and 25 percent in women.

Do you still doubt that the three major killers of Americans: heart disease, stroke, and cancer can be prevented simply by changing your way of life? A two-year study of 87,000 women and 45,000 men found that taking just one antioxidant, vitamin E, cut the risk of heart disease by 50 percent in women and by 25 percent in men. Women who ate five or more serving of carrots per month, which are high in the antioxidants vitamin A and beta carotene, had a 68 percent lower risk of stroke than women who had only one serving per month.

And, finally, in one of the most compelling studies on the relationship between lifestyle and degenerative disease, a two-decade study of more than 27,000 adult Seventh-Day Adventists, who adhere to a strict vegetarian diet and refrain from smoking and drinking, compared to the general population, found that adherents had lower rates of coronary heart disease and cancer, including colon cancer and, in women, ovarian cancer.

If we *choose* to exercise and we *choose* to eat properly and adequately supplement our diet, we are *choosing* to live a longer and healthier life.

THERE IS NO LIMIT TO LIFE-SPAN

The good-for-nothing Mediterranean fruit fly is finally good for something. It has shown us that the longer we live, the longer we can expect to live.

Normally, the medfly lives 20 to 30 days. But entomologist James Carey found that some medflies live three times that long and a tiny minority survive to 171 days—five to six times the normal life expectancy for that species. Carey and James Vaupel, a Duke University demographer, found that the older the flies were, the smaller their chances of dying on a given day (according to a standard mortality curve for that species.) When the medflies were 40 to 60 days old, their chance of dying decreased by 15 percent, and when they were 100 days or more, it fell to an astonishing four percent.

This research smashes the biological clock theory of aging,

i.e., the idea that there is a ticking bomb in our cells that controls aging and life-span. Says Carey: "If there were a clock, you'd expect that there would be an age where mortality rates would approach 100 percent. But our data clearly show that after a certain age, mortality rates actually level off and even decrease. That certainly supports the argument that there is no biological clock."

Believe it or not, what's true of the medfly is also true of humans. When Vaupel examined the impeccably kept records of Sweden's Lutheran Church for the past two centuries, he noted the same striking rate of decline in mortality rate in people over 100 years of age. He also discovered that, over the past 50 years, the mortality rate for the oldest of the old plunged by 17 percent for men and 33 percent for women. It now appears that a standard formula long used in insurance tables, the Gompertz curve, which shows that after age 30 the likelihood of dying doubles every seven years, does not apply to the oldest members of the population. So stick around, folks. The older we get, the better we do!

WHY STOP AT 100?

We need only look at history to see that very old people have not only survived, they have also prospered. Titian did some of his most beautiful paintings in his ninth decade; Michelangelo painted the breathtaking Sistine Chapel and wrote poetry until he died at 89; ancient Greek philosophers Socrates, Heraclitus, and Pythagoras (who gave us the theorem that tortured us in high school) lived a combined total of 285 years.

How can you still be laughing, loving, active, and living into your 90s and 100s? The how-to is simple: by arming yourself with knowledge. The lifestyle choices spelled out in the following chapters will enable you to dodge the bullets of disease and disability.

2

*"If wrinkles must be
written upon our brows,
let them not be written upon the heart.
The spirit should never grow old."*

JAMES A. GARFIELD

CHAPTER TWO

DON'T GROW OLDER, GROW BOLDER

Role Models and Successful Agers

It's one thing to be told how to age well; it's another to see it in action. The following people defy the stereotypes of aging, demonstrating that age (experience) has undeniable benefits that enhance life, encourage success, and can be very, very beautiful.

LIVING LONG IS THE BEST REVENGE

In 1965, Andre-Francois Raffay, a lawyer in southern France, had a bright idea. He agreed to pay 90-year-old Jeanne Calment of Arles, France, $500 a month for the right to inherit her apartment. It turned out to be a investment disaster. Not only did she outlive him, but by the time he passed on in 1995, he had paid her three times what the apartment was worth.

"Sorry I'm still alive," Madame Calment wrote him on her birthday as she did every year, "but my parents didn't raise shoddy goods." As previously mentioned, in August, 1997, when Calment died at the age of 122, she was the longest living person in the world.

George F. Abbott, playwright, director, actor, and producer, was a youthful 96 when he married his second wife, Joy, who was 40 years his junior. At 99, between rounds of golf, Abbott knocked out two new plays. At 102 he went on to co-direct one of those plays. He died at 107. His formula for aging was also very simple: "Have fun. And go home when you're tired."

Age has undeniable benefits that enhance life, encourage success, and can be very, very beautiful.

At 80 years of age, omni-energetic comedian Carol Channing shows off a 7-carat diamond ring and a radiant glow, thanks to a new fiancé. Career still flourishing, she is performing in the Broadway musical *Little Cupid*.

Some people feel old at 40, and others live young at 90. What makes the difference? Andre Maurois, the French essayist, biographer, and novelist who continued working into his 80s, observed that some people are just too busy to grow old. Meaningful activity, working hard, and having a purpose in life means looking forward to living every day of your life.

LIVING A PURPOSE-DRIVEN, VALUE-CENTERED LIFE

When Alice in Wonderland came to a fork in the road, she asked the Cheshire cat which road she should take. The cat asked, "Where are you going?" "I don't know," she said. The cat replied wisely, "If you don't know where you are going, any road will take you there."

A purpose-driven, value-centered life gives focus. It is the most life-enhancing, health-endowing, longevity-imparting characteristic one can have. We need to feel our lives have significance. In order to achieve significance we need to have an objective—a North Star—in our lives.

I have learned to give, enjoying blessings in return. Become a servant, a sower, and you will reap like kind. Don't waste your life's resources. God grants peace to those who serve a purpose.

By giving to others you will receive blessings money can't buy. Don't feel as though you don't or can't deserve prosperity and success. Help others achieve it, and you will see it for yourself.

Expecting to reap what you sow is not an abstract or selfish concept. It is an understanding of the law of the universe. When a farmer throws seed onto the earth, he expects a return on his investment. He expects a harvest that will more than compensate him for his efforts.

Every bite of food you ate today was brought about by sowing and reaping. All of life is based on this concept. It is a tried and true law of the universe.

Passion is the result of a focused life. Nothing in life is quite as powerful as a purpose-driven, value-centered life. Think what would have happened if Abraham Lincoln had gotten distracted. What if George Washington had decided it wasn't worth the trouble?

George Washington Carver, who died in 1943 at 79 years of age, focused on improving agriculture in the southern states of the U.S. He promoted growing peanuts and soybeans, which both restore nitrogen to the soil. This was important to the South because the exclusive cultivation of cotton and tobacco over many generations had impoverished the soil.

He saw the peanut as an alternative form of protein for very poor farmers. He saw the industrialization of the peanut as a way to free the black race from the hardships of the cotton industry.

This one value-centered, purpose-driven man, from 1923 to 1940, turned peanuts into the biggest cash crop in the South. He took the lowly peanut and turned it into 300 new products, including lipstick, soap, shampoo, shoe polish, paint, shaving cream, paper, imitation marble, dye, plastic, wood stain, etc. One value-centered, purpose-driven man touches our lives in real and useful ways daily. He declined a lucrative job promoting the peanut and refused to patent his discoveries, stating that because God had inspired them, they belonged to God, not him.

During the 1968 Olympics, it was the perseverance of one such value-centered, purpose-driven man, a Somalian Olympic runner by the name of John Stephen Akwahri, who came in an incredible three hours after the next to last runner. When he was asked why he persevered, he replied, "My country sent me here not just to run the race, but to finish the race."

Consider the postage stamp, my friend. It secures success through its ability to stick to one thing until it gets there. The difference between perseverance and obstinacy is that perseverance is born of a worthy goal.

The National Health Federation is the oldest and largest health freedom organization in America. I have served as its president for 17 years. The NHF is responsible for the freedom you now enjoy to purchase vitamins over the counter and for doctors to practice alternative healing. The war rages still, as we continue to educate, legislate, and litigate. To join the NHF in this noble battle call 1-800-993-2166.

We, like Thomas Paine, are pamphleteers. Horace Mann once said, "Be ashamed to die until you have won some victory for humanity." My tombstone will read, "America is freer because she lived." Every one of you has the right to put that on your tombstone.

Once people begin to see clearly why their work is worthwhile, big things can happen. What kind of big things? Well, it ranks right up there with love and hate. It's called self-esteem. In order to have self-esteem, it's not enough to have a well-understood and shared goal. It matters how you reach that goal. You must be guided by values. You have to be proud of both the goal and how you get there. I take no salary from the National Health Federation, pay all my own expenses, and donate monthly. To me, returning health and freedom to our people and vigor to our Nation is priceless.

A simple but inspirational and eloquent book entitled *Gung Ho!* by Ken Blanchard and Sheldon Bowles (William Morrow, N.Y., 1998) has words to learn by and values to hold in tough times. A truth of nature is one to remember, "Bad weather makes good wood."

"You can proclaim a value all you want, and you need to do that, but values become real only when you demonstrate them in the way you behave. Goals are set, but values are lived. Values are rocks you can count on. Rocks don't move in a swirling river, pebbles roll. Even if you call them rocks." From the book is a marvelous little poem I love.

"Hold or Roll" BY MANLY GRANT

Rocks hold firm while waters might
Sends pebbles rolling left and right
Call pebbles rock?
Set firm their goal?
First flash flood, still pebbles roll.
Not name, nor goal divide the two.
It's how they act. It's what they do.
Size dictates to stone, but you're in control.
Are you a rock or pebble?
Will you hold or roll?

I thank God each day for my purpose-driven life. I'm too busy to feel old, and I don't think about my chronological age. I am consumed by the fulfillment of my life's goals and my work. My work is my passion, and my purpose is to see to it that my message of illness-defying health transforms as many lives as possible.

Research is a constant adventure. Identifying the cause of someone's ill health is like solving a murder mystery. When I share my discoveries in books, articles, and on television, I feel God's pleasure.

I love seeing people's lives transformed daily—e.g.: the woman and man who were saved from the ravaging effects of multiple sclerosis; the Alzheimer's sufferer lifting the haze from his brain, enabling him to rejoin his family and resume his productive work as an insurance salesman; Linda, trapped in the downward spiral of Crohn's Disease, now enjoying health with a husband and two new children; Ann, who couldn't produce tots, has now borne three children; and the 6' 5" New York attorney who cried each day as he looked at his 5- and 7-year-old daughters because 12 doctors told him the final solution for his case of Lou Gehrig's disease would be death. He now lives a death-defying life.

I could go on and on and on. What a great honor it is to touch another person's life for the better! I thank God and am humbled by the anointing He has invested in my life. It has allowed me to know for certain that the law of reaping and sowing has not been repealed, for while directing my energies toward blessing the lives of others, I inadvertently heap blessings on my own.

Many have been blessed, thanks to their purpose-driven lives. Their achievements are inspirations to us all. Sir Edmund Hillary, the first man to climb Mount Everest, said he did it "because it was there." He did it because he knew that by challenging himself, he would improve himself. He did it because he knew he could do anything he set his mind to.

At the age of 110, Jeanne Calment was quoted as saying: "I had to wait 110 years to become famous. I intend to enjoy it as long as possible," and she did, for another 12 years.

We will now introduce you to men and women who have mastered the challenge of aging through dogged persistence, humor, an unquenching faith in God, and perhaps a little naivete.

ROLE MODELS OF SUCCESS

Success, achievement, and fulfillment have no age barriers. Rachel Torchia, who at 52 founded Gateway Title Agency lamented, "Most women in their 40s think that they are done and they know it all. It's a shame."

No matter how old you are or what condition you are in, you can and must change your life today, and if you do, all your tomorrows will be different.

If you ever find yourself saying "I'm too old to..." consider the following people who didn't stop trying.

At 50, Emily Post published her book *Etiquette*.

At 62, Colonel Harland Sanders started his franchise business, Kentucky Fried Chicken.

At 52, Ray Kroc started *his* franchise business, McDonald's.

At 80, John Huston directed the movie *The Dead*.

At 81, journalist I. F. Stone published the bestseller *The Trial of Socrates*, and daredevil Mary Victor Bruge flew a loop-the-loop 37 years after retiring from the cockpit.

At 83, Sidney Yates of Chicago began his 15th term in the U.S. Congress.

At 87, Mary Baker Eddy founded the *Christian Science Monitor*.

At 88, Doris Eaton Travis got a degree in history from the University of Oklahoma.

At 91, Hulda Crooks scaled Mount Whitney, the highest mountain in the continental U.S.

At 93, South Carolina Senator Strom Thurmond was declared the oldest person ever to serve in Congress. He holds U.S. Senate records for both the longest time served (since 1955) and the oldest Senator (born in 1902). He finished out his term of office at the age of 100.

In addition to the foregoing, there are those who transcend time; whose prolific lives and incredible accomplishments have been or will become immortalized.

The World Will Remember. . .

WORLD CAREGIVER EDDIE ALBERT

At over 90 years of age, my great friend Eddie Albert has become known for much more than his memorable role in the '60s sitcom *Green Acres*. Even if he wasn't my friend, he would still rank among my "most admired."

More than an image on television, the Broadway stage, and the movie screen, Eddie is an intelligent, personable man who deeply cares about the people and the world he lives in. He is committed to helping solve global problems of hunger, poverty, pollution, and soil erosion.

As the official representative of "Meals for Millions," a non-profit organization that provides food supplements to poor countries, he visited the late Albert Schweitzer to gain his wisdom and insights on malnutrition. This visit became part of a documentary that demonstrates the benefits of supplementation, and has been shown throughout the world.

In his fight against pollution, he helped dramatize the plight of California pelicans on Anacapa Island. They were unable to reproduce because insecticide residues had depleted their eggs of calcium.

Eddie has long been interested in nutrition and organic farming, and I have lunched from his amazing organic gardens. Having been introduced to vitamins more than 60 years ago by Dr. John H. Kellogg (the founder of Kellogg cereals), he is a staunch believer in the benefits of nutritional supplemention. His love and zest for life and healthy eating are evidenced by the tremendous vigor and energy that permeates everything he does. Eddie Albert is truly an ageless wonder.

MUSICAL STAR KATHRYN GRAYSON

Kathryn Grayson is one of my most cherished friends. She began her Hollywood career (at the age of 16) with the longest screen test in motion picture history. It included singing opera, pop music, and acting (both drama and comedy). Grayson went on to win everyone's heart with her sweet face and soaring soprano voice. Over the next 15 years, she appeared in 20 pictures, including such memorable musicals as *Showboat, Kiss Me Kate, Anchors Aweigh,* and *Ziegfield Follies.* She is a true Renaissance woman, with talent, beauty, and brains flowing from every pore.

Meaningful activity, working hard, and having a purpose in life means looking forward to living every day of your life.

Many of the early MGM studio divas turned to prescription uppers and downers to get them through their hectic, fast-paced careers, often becoming drug dependent. Kathryn did just the opposite. She ate healthy, got plenty of sleep, and took time off to rest.

Now in her 70s, she has successfully battled diabetes and has lost 35 pounds. She has all her own teeth; her skin is flawless—like porcelain; and she still has the four-range voice of an angel.

Today this energetic senior tours Australia in *Red Roses,* sings to packed houses at the London Palladium, and is a favorite in the Florida Keys, where she performs annual shows at the Show Boat. Her riveting appearances continue to dot the maps of three continents.

Kathryn has kept her beautiful voice meticulous. She shares the priceless wealth of her life experiences, proving her voice is stronger than ever by teaching voice classes at three universities.

Young people not familiar with Kathryn's musical legacy are discovering that, even in our later years, productivity and beauty need not be diminished, and creativity and inspiration can continue indefinitely.

CAROLYN CHANDLER—LEADER AND VISIONARY

Nothing in life is quite as powerful as a purpose-driven, value-centered life.

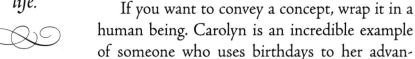

If you find yourself surveying the breathtaking San Francisco skyline, consider that almost every stellar property in San Francisco is managed by Chandler Properties. Even more remarkable is that the CEO, Carolyn Chandler, did it all by herself, through the force of her own will. At 56 years of age, she shows no signs of aging or slowing down.

If you want to convey a concept, wrap it in a human being. Carolyn is an incredible example of someone who uses birthdays to her advantage—struggling, striving, determined to improve her life with every year. Once you've seen and known the vibrancy, the carefully studied elegance of Carolyn, you can't help but agree the best is yet to come.

Carolyn spent her early years living in a one-room trailer with her mother and stepfather. She survived frequent moves and an unstable homelife by reading and searching out every new town's library and church. She knew what she was missing and was determined to learn how to get it. Through books and church teachings, she set out to improve her mind, spirit, and her life.

Carolyn Chandler is the epitome of the self-made woman. By the time she was 27, she was selling investment properties for Coldwell Banker Realty. At 35 she started her own real estate business, Chandler Properties, which bought, sold, and developed investment properties. In 1988, at age 44, she turned her focus to managing San Francisco's choicest condominiums.

Her recent corporate move is an analogy for successful aging. After 39 years of working both hard and smart, she promoted herself from Chief Operations Officer (daily management) to Chief Executive Officer. She sees herself not as a laborer or even a manager. Instead, she takes charge of her life as a leader and a visionary.

Carolyn's secrets to a life well-lived are having something to do, something to believe in, and someone to love. Carolyn loves her daughter Samantha totally and unselfishly, and has lavished her time, attention, and counsel on her.

Carolyn's confidence is built on the many difficulties she has overcome. "Without all these life experiences, I could never have achieved what I've achieved," she says. At 56 years young, Carolyn has it all. She welcomes the coming years for the new adventures and obstacles that offer opportunities to become more confident, competent, and impacting. Carolyn has been a positive influence on many lives, including mine, and she looks forward to new and rewarding challenges in the years to come.

BARBARA BROOKINS-SCHNEIDER — A SELF-MADE WOMAN IN A MAN'S WORLD

Defying the female stereotype of her time, Barbara Brookins-Schneider not only excelled in corporate finance but crashed through the glass ceiling for herself and others to follow.

When her father died at 16, she accepted the challenge to pave her own way and joined the workforce. Putting her exquisite photographic memory and an incredible aptitude for math to work, she began by handling accounts receivable in a credit office.

"I had to learn discipline at an early age. I had to make grown-up decisions," she said. At 18 she received a scholarship to attend college but was held back from her dream of being an aeronautical engineer because Cal Tech would not accept women into its undergraduate program.

Determined to either find a way or make one, she continued her education at Occidental College and obtained a B.A. in economics with a specialization in finance at UCLA. College wasn't easy. She knew she would be disappointed if she failed at her endeavor, but would be doomed if she didn't try. And try she did. In addition to her college work, she held down three jobs to survive and pay tuition.

After graduation, Barbara entered a world dominated by men and fierce competition. (No, not sports.) In 1962, at a time when few women were in finance, she became a registered stockbroker at Shearson Hammill. In 1966, at the age of 26, she became an institutional stockbroker—one of only three women in the country. As highly competitive as her world was, she knew that if the clients she served realized financial success, it would reflect positively on her and her company. She distinguished herself by working harder, working smarter, and never expecting deferential treatment. She led with her strengths, remembering that dressing well and being well-groomed is the first thing people notice and that charm and conciliation solve many a problem.

At 40 years of age, Barbara became the head of a savings and loan, working 16- to 18-hour days seven days a week. She honed her organizational skills working with regulators, investors, and a predominately male board of directors. At this turning point in her life, she said, "I learned that I could devote myself solely to the business at hand and solve problems and resolve crises, and that, "Nothing is work unless you'd rather be doing something else."

In the late '70s, Barbara founded, funded, and opened San Francisco-based Pyramid Savings and Loan (now East West Bank) as Chairman of the Board and President, leaving behind the men who scoffed, "Why should you make as much money as I do?" She excelled financially at a time when primarily men were allowed to earn money, and women were denied equal opportunity for success. But something was missing. She wasn't achieving as much as she knew she could.

Barbara almost lost it all when her health declined as the stress of her responsibilities increased. She looked in the mirror, saw herself aging prematurely, and realized that without her health, her financial success didn't mean a thing. Without skipping an ambitious beat, she poured time into turning herself around.

First she set out to educate herself. She read my book *Foods That Heal* cover to cover and subscribed to the National Health Federation's magazine, *Health Freedom News*. She learned which minerals and vitamins to take, exercised passionately, and, thanks to better health, became more efficient with her time. She didn't work less, she worked better. With renewed health and well-being, she found she accomplished more in less time.

The difference between perseverance and obstinacy is that perseverance is borne of a worthy goal.

Today, her health and beauty are traits others admire. Working as hard on herself as her business, she exercises every morning, alternating fast aerobic walking with yoga and weight training. When she travels she walks or finds a gym.

Barbara continues to keep up on the most current nutritional information, never missing a copy of *Health Freedom News* and reading my newest book *All Your Health Questions Answered Naturally*.

Barbara knows that diet and rest are vitally important. She eats chemical-free fresh wild game for her protein source and plenty of vegetables. She eats meals no less than three and no more than five hours apart, snacking on vegetables, eating dinner early, and going to bed early, making sure to get eight or nine hours of sleep.

Barbara is in her early 60s and refuses to "retire," choosing instead to devote her life to charitable causes, enjoy financial independence, and supporting others to do the same.

Barbara is setting up a foundation to help aspiring young women who, like she, have brains, talent, and acumen. She wants to make sure they have the financial resources to achieve their potential. Determined to preserve classical music for the next generation, she is a generous supporter and volunteer for the symphony.

"My joy is in watering and fertilizing these young minds and watching them grow. We grow from sharing our bounty," she says.

MARTI MCMAHON—IMMIGRANT ENTREPRENEUR

There is a reason people from all over the world want to come to America. It's the land of opportunity. But what many forget is that success in America requires hard work, dedication, and taking advantage of opportunities when they present themselves.

Marti McMahon was four-year-old Marti Cornejo when her family came to Chicago from El Salvador, Central America. They had little money, but lots of love and a desire to work. At age 7, Marti's mother taught her how to make flowers from tissue and, eager to help with the family finances, Marti sold her flowers door to door for 50 cents apiece.

"My mother was creative and talented," Marti remembers. "It was from her that I learned to recycle, before it was fashionable to do so. When I was 11 she had an alteration-dressmaking store in the basement of our apartment building. She made all my clothes and taught me about fabric, colors, painting, and upholstery, setting the groundwork for the creativity I would need for my future business endeavors."

At 22 years of age, Marti started a fashion design business in Chicago. She was in her 40s when she transformed one dilapidated boat into a yacht, while raising three small children by herself. She was getting older, but no less bolder.

A fleet of ships followed, lovingly refurbished by Marti's hands and expertise. She turned her personal love of yachting, entertaining, and gourmet cooking into the Bay Area's premier luxury yacht charter service. Pacific Marine Yachts has earned many Bay Area business awards, including Top 100 Fastest Growing Bay Area Companies (1993), Best of Show for presentation at the 1998 American Culinary Federation Show, and Bay Area's 100 Largest Woman-Owned Businesses 1994-1998. Her personal business prowess was celebrated when Marti earned "Woman Entrepreneur of the Year" by the San Francisco Chamber of Commerce in 1989.

"If I had not had the skills of a do-it-yourselfer, Pacific Marine Yachts could not have happened," Marti testifies. "I wanted to show my kids that no matter what happens, you can make it if you save your money and work hard."

Pacific Marine is now Signature Yachts, owned by Marti's daughter and son-in-law. Marti continues her involvement as the company's investor and promoter, staying active and ageless.

Marti credits her hard work and youthful philosophies with keeping herself young and energetic. Defeating age with attitude, Marti accepts problems as challenges and uses creativity to find positive solutions; finding joy in keeping the mind, spirit, and body active and fulfilled, seeking change as an essential part of life and envisioning a future of possibilities.

Marti views life as a gift from God, and each day brings her a sense of adventure. This is evident in her determination to push herself physically. She hits the gym at 7 A.M. each morning for one hour of aerobics, then an hour of weight training. When we ski together, I see firsthand the secret to her youthfulness: her courage to dare, the openness to blaze new trails, and the passionate joy she brings to each new endeavor.

SOPHIA LOREN—ETERNAL BEAUTY

In April of 1995, at the opening of the San Francisco Museum of Art, I had the great good fortune to meet legendary Italian film star Sophia Loren and her husband, producer Carlo Ponti. While her curvaceous body couldn't be ignored, I was taken by the fact that she was even more beautiful close up. Although everyone was bidding for her attention, when we spoke, she fixed her enormous green eyes on me as if I were the only person in the room.

You can defeat age with an attitude of accepting problems as challenges and using your creativity to find positive solutions.

"How did you arrive at age 60 looking like you do?" I asked her. "Determination, dedication, and discipline," she replied. "Where do those characteristics come from?" I wanted to know. "It comes from within," she said. "Nobody can teach them to you."

Then I asked her what her secrets were. "There are no secrets," she told me. "You must start out each day anew expecting wonderful things to happen to you. That doesn't happen by accident. You set your own mindset. That's how character is developed."

When I asked how she retains her beauty, glamour, and sex appeal, she said, "I think what you have inside reflects very much in your face, in your expression. If you can find a kind of equilibrium in life, you never really get old because you have that kind of ingenuity and innocence inside that gives you that brightness and that glint in your eye that generally, getting older, you lose."

She maintains her figure by exercising every morning, stretching, and doing abdominals for 45 minutes every day. She eats well, but in moderation.

She doesn't jog or do aerobics because her famous breasts get in the way. Laughing, she says, "I have to hold my two things."

Sophia lifts light weights of half a kilo (a little over a pound) but is gradually lifting heavier weights. "I'm going to become a superwoman with oil on my muscles," she jokes.

To maintain her gorgeous complexion, she keeps her skin clean and nourished by "eating the right things. The mirror of your health is your skin," she says. "If you drink, it shows on your face. If you eat the wrong foods you have pimples. If you take care of yourself and you lead a healthy life, your skin will look wonderful."

When asked how she feels about getting older, she answers truthfully, "I can't tell you that I like it, but I think I can cope with it because everybody gets older. Sometimes it's a little upsetting because time goes by and you want to do more, and you have to accept life for what it is and find some new motivation that gives you drive and enthusiasm."

But then, almost without realizing it, she imparts a secret of eternal youth. "You can always dream. Life is full of dreams that you can fulfill. When I'm walking along in the street, I always feel that around the corner there is something wonderful waiting for me. That's my attitude. You really have to be satisfied with what you are and accept from life what it still very generously offers you—and notice it, and be glad for it."

GEORGE FOREMAN—THE COMEBACK KID

A lot of world-class athletes are trying to break the hardest record of all—the age barrier. And I don't mean ageism. I'm talking about clearing the hurdles of decreasing maximum oxygen output, loss of muscle mass, and the mindset that says at a particular age—it differs from sport to sport—you're history. Your number is up on the wall, not on your back.

Age gave a knockout punch to youth when George Foreman,

three months shy of his 46th birthday, floored 26-year-old Michael Moorer to become heavyweight champion of the world, 20 years after Foreman last held the title. Nearly everyone was counting the old fighter out before the fight began, calling him too soft, too fat, too old. They predicted a rout and it was—for Foreman.

Other notable sports figures have competed against aging. Sugar Ray Leonard, 38, said it was not the money that motivated his comebacks, but that he "needed the arena." He enjoys the recognition, respect, and near reverence that come from his victories in the ring.

Olympic seven-gold medal swimmer Mark Spitz at 41, five-time Wimbledon tennis champion Bjorn Borg at 34, and Hall of Fame pitcher Jim Palmer at 45 all tried comebacks with varying degrees of success.

Michael Jordan, at age 38, after a two-year hiatus, is making a miraculous comeback in the National Basketball League. He is still an effective player who can dominate opponents who were babies when he began his professional career.

As we learn to take care of our bodies and throw off the yoke of ageism, we can enjoy sports later in life. In 1998, about 4.5 million American men aged 35 to 44 were still playing basketball, according to a report by the Sporting Goods Manufacturers Association, nearly double from the previous decade, when only 2.5 million American men aged 35 to 44 were actively playing basketball.

As long as we keep ourselves healthy, only our beliefs keep us from participating in sports. While skiing the slopes of Mt. Rose, Nevada, I met a man who not only demonstrates this every day on a personal level, but teaches it to others. His name is Rusty Crook. He is 68 years old, a former U.S. Olympic Ski Team coach and former Olympic speed skater who teaches seniors how to ski.

Rusty has taught his older students that they need not be limited by their expectations and despite their advanced years can hang glide, snowboard, and ski with the best of them. I watched an 84-year-old pupil confidently swoop down the slopes like a teenager, and other seniors have learned it's never too late to try snowboarding and hang gliding.

He has shown me and others that our liabilities are limitations of the mind only, and that if we only try we may be very surprised at what we can accomplish. As Rusty's training boosts his students' confidence, courage, and self-esteem, it breaks down stereotypes, leading the way for the next generation to enjoy life longer.

Even if you're not a world-class athlete and your Olympic dream is limited to getting a pair of tickets to the figure skating finals, you can make your own personal comeback. Don a pair of skis, put on roller skates, pick up a tennis racket or a golf club.

One of the best things you can do for yourself is get a good comfortable pair of walking shoes, grab your spouse, dog, kids, or significant other and go for a good long walk.

Walking is a very beneficial exercise and almost everyone can do it. It also gives opportunities for learning and new perspectives on where you are. Recently, I hiked all over Lisbon, Portugal, then Paris. I realized that although I have been to both cities before, I never really experienced them.

Learn a new sport, master an old one, compete at your age and skill level. You will not only benefit your body, mind, and spirit, you will give age the boot and feel young all over again.

LOIS LEHRMAN—SELLING KNOWLEDGE

With her blonde hair and deep blue eyes, Lois Lehrman is a vision of beauty, strength, and power. The image you perceive of her from the outside was born from within. She was a single mother with two young children to support when she took her first sales job in the male-dominated life insurance industry.

"A good appearance gets you in the door," she said, "But you must quickly establish your knowledge." Lois soon realized if she could sell insurance she could sell anything. So long as she could sell, she would always have something that was valuable to other people.

From insurance she went into the newspaper business in New Jersey selling advertising and literally putting small papers on the map. In her 50s she moved to San Francisco and spotted a small social paper with good potential that had failed to turn a profit. Although she was 55 at the time, she decided to buy the paper as a way of ensuring self-employment until she chose to retire. Under Lehrman's management, *The Nob Hill Gazette* has grown enormously in both distribution and appeal.

She says, "I find that being busier than I've ever been in my life has made me less concerned about aging," and she forgets how old she is until she takes a long look in the mirror. Being in the newspaper business has "expanded my horizons," and also expanded her circle of friends, from her daughters' peers (in their 30s) to people in their 90s. Her friends come from every walk of life and every corner of the world.

Successful aging, she discovered, is "finally being comfortable with myself. I like being 100 percent involved in a business," and she is gratified that she continues to earn enough income to safeguard her future. Lois may be aging chronologically, but she insists "I'm still working on what I want to be when I grow up."

SUSAN BLAIS—DARE TO DREAM

My friend Susan Blais has shown me that I may dare to dream. Her creativity and enterprise have taken her from hardship to prosperity, and have helped many others prosper as well.

Susan was just 19, living in Oregon, when she married. She and her husband bought a house for $4,000, renovated it, and sold it. When she was 20 they bought another house. At 25, her husband left her with four preschool children. Regarding her shocking loss she told me, "I had no choice but to win. I had my children to think of."

In order to provide stability for her chidren, she refinanced her house and bought a farm. She sustained the farm by share-cropping, i.e., leasing the land to farmers to grow their crops. She subsequently subdivided the acreage and took her children to live in the sunshine of California. There she began selling real estate.

After the big Los Angeles earthquake, Susan witnessed the loss of entire neighborhoods. Tenements and apartment build-ings were abandoned, boarded up and in ruins. Drug dealers and squatters moved in, and the neighbors feared for their lives. Now in her mid 50s, Susan knew she had to do something.

She wanted to recharge the energy of the neighborhoods, help them bring back their self-respect. She did exactly that. She bought abandoned buildings and refurbished them with style, charm, warmth. . .and history. Confronted with Susan's resolve, criminals fled the neighborhoods. Now her buildings are 100 percent occupied and are thriving residences for their inhabi-tants.

"QUEEN OF THE FUNDRAISERS" BELLA FARROW

"The Queen of Nob Hill," "The Diva of Fund Raisers," the exuberant, irrepressible barely five-foot-tall Bella Farrow is San Francisco's best known fundraiser.

In a city renowned for its great opera, symphony, and ballet, Bella reigns. For the past 40 years, this irrepressible, energetic matriarch has overcome life-threatening surgery and the effects of time by doing what she loves best—getting people to part with their money for charitable and noble causes. In 1995, she was named San Francisco's *Woman of the Year*. In 1999, she was appointed to the board of trustees of the San Francisco Performing Arts.

Though Bella is old enough to remember the Great Depression, men young and old still seek her out, waiting in line to squire her. She is sought by anyone who wants to add life to their party or event.

Because I'm close to her I know the rigors of Bella's schedule and am astonished at her stamina and energy. She attends a party, luncheon, or event every single day. She knows so many people that everywhere she goes she is greeted by someone. She radiates a spirit of indomitable energy that not only embraces people to her, but melts away her seven-plus decades.

With so many fundraising events and social engagements, you would expect her to have an assistant or secretary. Even at 80 years old, she writes every invitation by hand and does everything herself with an old-fashioned Rolodex.

Bella is so popular and successful that people flock to be in her company. She is the hostess of the annual charity event, Girls Town of Italy fashion show and luncheon held at the Fairmont Hotel in San Francisco. She not only gets world famous designers like Nolan Miller and Mark Zunino to participate, but because her name is associated with the event, every year a record number of people fork over $175 each to have lunch and participate.

To stay young and age well, she advises people to "GET INVOLVED." (You can hear the capital letters in her voice.) "If you get involved in doing things for others, you'll find that in the long run, it'll be doing things for you." Her dark eyes spark home the depth of her convictions. Bella suggests that people volunteer in their church, various charities, or local politics. "Keep yourself busy, your mind busy, your body busy, and then you can receive the best benefits of all, which are good emotional and physical health."

Keeping herself physically active is also on Bella's agenda for a long life. She scales the San Francisco hills daily, opting to walk instead of calling a cab. Healthy eating means she chooses a salad with plain vinegar dressing and never indulges in dessert.

BARBARA CARTLAND—LIFE, LESSONS, AND LOVE

Barbara Cartland was the queen of romance writers, a woman as renowned for her productivity as her pronouncements on "living young, looking young, and being beautiful inside and out." She was energized by her work and embraced the youthful attributes of her romantic heroines.

Cartland's legacy includes advice on aging well. She would say that "age begins in the brain. If one thinks old, one becomes old. Keep your brain active and take an intelligent interest in new ideas, new projects, and new activities." She called it fatal "to let (older people) think they are out-of-date, unwanted, and an encumbrance," emphasizing work. "When I look around at the enormous number of people I know all over the world, I find it is not those who are rich who are happy—it is those who are working," she said. "The joy of life, what the French call joie de vivre, comes from developing the brain."

Cartland lived on a 400-acre estate near London, produced 6,000 to 7,000 words in an average afternoon and, according to her publicist, she could write an entire book in seven of those afternoons. Sales, in 36 languages, of her 723 books exceeded one billion copies worldwide.

Cartland died at age 98, leaving behind a legacy of popular books and models for postponing age through productivity.

ANN AND ROSCOE BEARD—A LIFETIME OF GIVING

Retiring after more than 50 years as ministers, Roscoe Beard and his wife, Ann, continue ministering on a volunteer basis, Ann at a nursing home and Roscoe at a prison. Staying active "keeps us young," says Ann, who at age 80 also waits on tables at a senior center three times a week and stuffs envelopes as part of a Retired Volunteer Senior Program.

They are dedicated to marriage and to each other, bearing in mind "the commitment we made on our wedding day." Part of their commitment to each other is to maintain their health. They abstain from smoking, drinking, and junk food, and try to maintain a balanced diet with lots of fresh fruits and vegetables. To retain the nutritional value of their food, they like to steam or pressure-cook the vegetables or eat raw yellow squash, broccoli, and zucchini in salad. They also supplement their diet with vitamins E, C, and plenty of minerals. The Beards combine exercise and socializing with friends by walking in a local shopping mall two miles three times a week, and, when they can't get out, do laps in their swimming pool. Most of all, they practice their faith. "Our confidence is in the Lord," Ann calls it.

They like to point out the advantages of growing older. "We can be an example to young people and help them because of what we have learned through life."

Their formula for staying young is to keep body and mind healthy and active, have a goal in life, and strive to meet it. "We keep our desires and longings before us." As always, their thoughts are for others. "Our priorities in life are to help others as much as we can and live so that we can hear Him say, 'Well done ye good and faithful servants.'"

THE REVEREND KENNY FOREMAN— PROMOTING FAMILY LIFE

At the age of seven, as Kenny lay dying of rheumatic fever, doctors told his mother there was no hope. Believing in God more than doctors, his mother solicited the power of prayer from friends and family. Kenny recovered.

Today, Kenny is celebrating 50 years of preaching the gospel. Through his multicultural Cathedral of Faith church, he inspires the hearts of 10,000-15,000 members.

Not content to help only his own parishioners, Kenny built a 30,000-square-foot Family Life Center that temporarily houses homeless families, helping them get back on their feet. Kenny joined the State of California in a project in which 30 troubled kids were brought to the Family Life Center for hope and education. All were successful in completing their high school education—their grades have consistently gone from Ds to Bs—and are expected to go on to live successful and productive lives.

When asked why he would take on such a huge endeavor at the age of 70, Kenny responded, "I never want to outlive my dreams."

Kenny inspires thousands, myself included. He, his wife, Shirley, and his family are truly the most loving people I know. Whether rich or poor, fashion-setter or street person, Kenny loves each member of the congregation unconditionally. Let's close this chapter with a gift from Kenny to you: his inspirational words.

Kenny Foreman's Four Secrets of Successful Living at Any Age: Perspective, Priority, Power, and Purpose

The four secrets of successful living at any age are perspective, priority, power, and purpose.

1. "You need a perspective to live from. Your problems are not as important as how you look at them. Because I know all things are working together for my good, I rejoice. God has a purpose behind every one of my problems.

2. "You need a priority to live by. Distinguish the trivial from the significant. You decide what is important. Focus on what counts, what really matters. In all things, put God before you, and He will reward you with success.

3. "Life can drain you. You need a fresh power supply to live on. With the help of the Holy Spirit you can be ready for anything, equal to everything.

CHAPTER THREE

SOCIAL SECURITY

How Love, Friendship, and Religion Extend Life

They're not related by blood, they're there by choice. They pay no heed if the dishes are still in the sink, but they notice immediately if you have a new haircut. They listen sympathetically, may offer too much advice, and often ignore your own. They are, by turns, petty, solicitous, infuriating, wonderful. But the truth is, we can't live without social attachments.

IN THIS CHAPTER, I WILL SHOW HOW GOD, friends, lovers, pets, family, and community, our vital connections to one another, enhance, enrich, and extend our lives.

Isolation is toxic to longevity, while intimacy and togetherness are a fistful of nutrients. Studies show that, on average, lonely people die younger, while relationships with others extend life.

One study on the benefits of social interaction involved 232 elderly patients who underwent heart surgery. Those who had the strongest participation in social groups had three times the survival rate of those who did not. This benefit was quite apart from the three-fold survival rate increase seen among people in the same study who found strength in religious faith. Nor does the kind of group matter, whether it is a church supper group, seniors club, or fraternal group. It appears that it is life protective to belong to a group and participate in regular social activity of any kind.

FINANCIALLY REWARDING

Here's a new twist to the old adage—It's not what you know, it's *who* you know. Cultivating your co-workers is a key to success. Even in such non-people-oriented fields as engineering, technical knowledge accounts for about 15 percent of earning power, while one's personality and skill in human engineering—the ability to handle people—account for the other 85 percent. This is according to studies by the Carnegie Institute of Technology.

In contrast to the foregoing, being fired is more often due to lack of social know-how than job performance. Researchers found that up to 80 percent of people were dismissed because they could not get along with their co-workers, while approximately 20 percent were let go because they could not do the job.

LOVE AND LOSS

Recently, a friend of mine spent a "perfect romantic evening" with an old flame she hadn't seen in 17 years. They had both been through a traumatic marriage and divorce. Now that they were both single, the man saw no reason why they couldn't resume their relationship. "I don't know," said my friend. "We had a wonderful time, and I feel exactly the same way I did about him 17 years ago. But part of me says, 'Don't get involved. Don't ruin something as perfect as it is now.'"

Now there's a solution to ending a relationship—don't start it. Or as a business executive, transferred dozens of times from one location to another, put it: "We've discovered that to prevent the pain of saying goodbye we no longer say hello."

The truth is, relationships are a lot like exercise—no pain, no gain. Loss is part of life, whether it is from death, separation, or the end of love. But even if it ends badly, leaving a seemingly irreparable scar on your heart, you'll still have had the experience of knowing that other person. Not to have known what it is like to love, cherish, and be deeply intimate with another person is the greatest loss of all.

PRESCRIPTION FOR HAPPINESS

In many different ways, Jesus said the way to find ourselves is to lose ourselves. You can't chase happiness. You can only let it catch up to you when you are lost in the giving of yourself. The way to win friends is not by making yourself the focus of attention, but by letting others know you care. Risk showing your feelings and talking about your affection. It can take many forms: a phone call, a note, a compliment, a bouquet of flowers, a book, or CD by someone that person likes—small messages of love that say, "I'm thinking of you."

As Ben Franklin said, "Speak ill of no man, but speak all the good you know of everybody." Praise is a gift you can freely bestow on others, and it comes back to you manyfold. The great cellist, Pablo Cassals, said, "As long as one can admire and love, then one is young forever."

GIVE YOUR FRIENDS SPACE

Relationships of any kind—between a man and a woman, a parent and child, or just close friends—are a balancing act between intimacy and independence. It is not enough to love, you must love freely. There are two things a parent can give a child—roots and wings. The same might be said of any nourishing relationship. At the heart of love there is a simple secret: the lover lets the beloved be free.

In interviews with hundreds of couples, married, living together, or divorced, researchers George and Nena O'Neill found that what people wanted most was a relationship *and* freedom.

While these desires may seem mutually exclusive, and contradictory, the best friendships and marriages do fulfill both needs. Think about the couples that you know. Is one partner usually silent while the other usually does most of the talking? Do their conversations consist mainly of put-downs? Do they speak proudly about the other person and use terms of encouragement? What characteristics do you notice about couples you know who are the happiest? Do they look into each other's eyes when they speak? Have they anticipated each other's needs? Does she fix something different for him (or ask you as their hostess to please his preference)? Are they considerate with each other in small things? Is there commonality of shared ideas? This requires depth of conversation. Is there commonality in the things they do? Do they ski together, golf together, play bridge, dance, and cook together? Do they go to the same church together? Do they touch (especially hug) each other? As a hostess, I ask my guests around the table to share, one by one, what they would like to be remembered for. What would they want written on their tombstone? The couples with the best marriages consistently express a desire to please their wife or husband.

God, friends, lovers, pets, family, and community, our vital connections to one another, enhance, enrich, and extend our lives.

KEEP TALKING

Talk is cheap, but you'd never guess it from the way most people act. How much time do you think the average couple spends talking to each other in the course of a week? If you guessed an hour a day, even a half hour a day, you're way off the mark. They spend all of 17 minutes. All that time just to decide who takes out the garbage!

A single-woman friend of mine asked me if I could fix her up with someone. "What kind of person do you have in mind?" I asked. "I don't care what he looks like or what he does," she said. "As long as he talks."

Conversation is the glue of relationships, even sexual ones. Even if you're not good at small talk, you can learn to excel in the art of intimacy. Here are a few simple rules:

1. **The road to the heart is the ear.** It's great to be sparkling, witty, well-informed, and impress others with your mind. But nothing is more interesting to another person than someone who is truly interested in them.

2. **Make eye contact.** When you're really involved in what someone says, you fasten your eyes on that person. The eye talk between you says, "At this moment in time, you are the only one in the world for me." Lia Belli is one of the most fascinating women I know, a woman with hundreds of friends all over the world. All of English society has fallen prey to my friend's personal power. She is the master of "the look," and while I have never caught her doing so, I swear she practices the look. Lia now lives in Romania with her husband, Prince Paul.

Observe how a flirting couple look at each other. Prolonged eye contact is the most important courting gesture in Western culture.

3. **Be stingy with advice.** One of the biggest mistakes we can make in conversation is to assume that when someone asks us for advice, he or she really means it. What they really want—and need—in most cases is a friendly listener. By allowing them to speak their mind and share their feelings, you often help them make their own decision about what should be done. This is

especially true in dealing with young people, who often are easily overwhelmed by too much advice from their elders.

4. **Safeguard secrets.** Trust is the basis of deep friendships. A woman friend told me about a shady incident in her past, prefacing her story by saying, "I'm trusting you with my life." When people confide their fears and secrets, they need reassurance that you won't think less of them. It is a great honor to be privy to information with which you could harm your friend. If you freely show your gratitude, you will open the way for greater intimacy. My dear friend Heide Betz is an Olympic champ at this technique. It is such a consistent standard of her character that it has won her the respect of everyone from San Francisco to London.

5. **Close the conversation loop.** Communication takes place when two conversational arcs form a circle. Silence, noncommittal grunts, and/or changing the subject keep the circle from closing. A woman who divorced her husband after ten years of marriage told me, "I felt like everything I said disappeared into a black hole." Often, all that is needed is a smile, a nod, a murmur of assent, which says, "I hear you, I know what you're saying." Attentive listening *is* the biggest ego booster.

A woman who lived during the Victorian era had the great fortune to dine, on consecutive nights, with two of the most distinguished prime ministers in British history, William Gladstone and Benjamin Disraeli.

"When I left the dining room after sitting next to Mr. Gladstone," she said, "I thought he was the cleverest man in England. But after sitting next to Mr. Disraeli, I thought I was the cleverest woman in England." Disraeli had the social talent to make others feel good about themselves. It no doubt greatly enhanced his popularity.

HEALTHY EMOTIONS

When you meet someone new, the topics are superficial: "Nice day today." "Do you think it will flood this winter?" When you get to know the person a bit better, you venture an opinion or two. "The state needs better flood control." When you really trust the person, you let your emotions show, and then it's a whole new ball game.

Isolation is toxic to longevity, while intimacy and togetherness are a fistful of nutrients.

Being able to freely express your feelings to another human being is one of life's great joys. There is a series of sculptures called "the prisoners." They were carved by the divinely inspired Michelangelo, and these statues seem to be struggling to emerge from the marble. They remind me of the difficulty that many people encounter as they struggle to express themselves and emerge as whole human beings.

Don't make the mistake of confusing emotion with weakness and stoicism with strength. The strong, silent type is enshrined in American books and movies. That's fine if you need John Wayne leading a cavalry charge, but it's cold comfort when what you need is a shoulder to cry on.

Communication is the mainstay of trust, honor, and faith; important traits by which to live a long and healthy life.

TEARS ARE GOOD FOR HEALTH

Why are alcoholics predominately male? In part, says California psychiatrist Taz W. Kinney, because men hate to cry. The tears we shed when we are sad or touched are different molecularly from the tears induced by peeling onions or a cold wind. Charles Dickens instinctively understood this when he wrote in

Oliver Twist, "crying opens the lungs, washes the countenance, exercises the eyes, and softens down the temper, so cry away."

And don't worry that your tears mark you as being vulnerable and needy. Nothing is quite as irresistible as a friend or lover who says, "I need you." Sharing our pain is one of life's greatest gifts. Shared joy is double joy, and shared sorrow is half-sorrow.

OWNING YOUR ANGER

They were one of the nicest couples I had ever met—friendly, warm, eager to please, like two young puppies. Then one day, rather abruptly, the woman walked out on her husband. "I don't understand it," he said to me. "We never had a fight." In other words, they never let each other know how they really felt.

Anger (just like every other emotion) cries out to be expressed. Some people fight dirty. They are passively hostile, suffering in silence or making snide remarks. Suppressed anger corrodes a relationship like rust in a drainpipe.

Another characteristic of suppressed anger is that it can build up a head of steam, erupting when you least expect it. "What are you so mad at?" we'll ask our mate when he or she blows up over who left the milk out all the night. Chances are the milk is just a diversion for something else that's going on, such as stress at work or an unresolved problem in the marriage.

Anger is not a negative emotion when it is expressed appropriately. It can be a driving force for creativity or stirring other people to action. "Men and motorcars progress by a series of internal explosions," wrote Channing Pollock.

PICK YOUR BATTLES

"An inexhaustible good nature is one of the most precious gifts of heaven, spreading itself like oil over the

troubled sea of thought, and keeping the mind smooth
and equable in the roughest weather."
WASHINGTON IRVING

Making and keeping friends requires tolerance, patience, and a good nature. Be tolerant of others' obvious weaknesses, foibles, and inadequacies. Your friend is always late and sometimes stands you up. But she is also insecure and sensitive. Do you address your frustration to her, or accept that aspect of her personality without complaint? People enjoy a good-natured person, one who lets the little problems slide without a second glance, and who appreciates the good things with enthusiasm. Have you ever known someone with a great sense of humor, who made you laugh? You wanted to be around him or her, didn't you? Because good-natured people are easy to be around, they have the most friends and invite the most acquaintances. Practice overcoming frustration without expressing displeasure. The conflict will pass, and you'll be glad you weren't the one to make it worse.

Not to have known what it is like to love, cherish, and be deeply intimate with another person is the greatest loss of all.

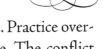

DON'T GIVE UP

People often complain that as they get older it is harder to make new friends. Most of the time it's because they just don't try in the same way they did when they were younger. The characteristics of youth include impetuousness, bravado, and naive confidence. As with anything else you want in life, you have to go after it not once, but many times over.

Don't let rejection get you down, because the next time you may connect. Babe Ruth hit 714 home runs, a record that stood for 40 years. But does anyone remember that he struck out 1,330 times, an all-time "low"? When asked the secret of his success, the Sultan of Swat said: "I just keep goin' up there and keep swingin' at 'em."

You don't fail until you quit trying.

A HUG A DAY

Here's a simple prescription for health and happiness: A hug, administered daily, or as often as you wish. A heartfelt hug is amazingly therapeutic. It can reduce stress, diminish anger, strengthen relationships, banish loneliness, and restore our faith in the world. Research points to the fact that people need human touch to feel their best, both emotionally and physically. Hugs can even counteract the negative effects that anger and tension have on the body, such as increased heart rate, blood pressure, and muscle tightness.

A CAUTIONARY TALE

In the foothills of the Blue Mountains of Pennsylvania there is a town called Roseto. It was settled in 1882 primarily by immigrants from a small town in Italy. For decades, the residents retained the traditions of their old country, marrying within their own ethnic group, living in three-generation households, attending church regularly, participating in social organizations, looking out for their neighbors. They appeared to live charmed lives.

In the early 1960s, two researchers, Stewart Wolf, M.D. and John G. Bruhn, came to town to try to discover why the death rate in Roseto was significantly lower than in three surrounding communities and the country as a whole. They looked at every aspect of the residents' lives. They found the citizens of Roseto ate the same amounts of meat and animal fat, smoked, and exercised as little as those living in neighboring towns.

After a five-year study, they came up with only one explanation for the residents' remarkable survival: the extraordinary close-knit ties of the residents to family and community. However, Wolf predicted, the trend toward "Americanization" would inevitably lead to a higher incidence of heart attacks.

Thirty years later, when the two researchers visited the town as part of a follow-up study, the loss of social cohesion in the community was striking. Residents married outside the "clan," became much more material, and abandoned their religious customs.

The change in lifestyle was epitomized by a couple who were living in a "big garish house" on the town's outskirts. Proudly, the woman showed off all the electric conveniences that made life easier.

But what she missed most, she said, was that no one ever dropped by for coffee. Where she used to live, she said, "There was always someone in my kitchen."

The people of Roseto are now no different from anyone else in the country, says Wolf, whose prediction, sadly, came to pass. The residents cleaned up their diets, cut down on dairy and animal fats, but their death rate from heart attacks rose until it is now the same or even higher than the national average.

In all likelihood few of us would want to live with our in-laws. And, goodness knows, someone dropping by unannounced for coffee could ruin a whole afternoon. But the next time you think you're too busy to pick up the phone and say "hello" to a friend, remember the price the Rosetoans paid for becoming just like their fellow citizens.

"SAY TWO PRAYERS AND CALL ME IN THE MORNING"

"Ask and it shall be given you; seek, and ye shall find; knock, and it shall be opened unto you:

For every one that asketh receiveth;
and he that seeketh findeth;
and to him that knocketh it shall be opened."
MATTHEW 7:7,8

Prayer is the most powerful medicine in the world. It doesn't require a prescription, costs absolutely nothing, is totally free of side effects, and is available any time, day or night. The vast majority of us take it on a regular basis. According to a 1992 cover story in *Newsweek*, 91 percent of women and 85 percent of men pray.

A fascinating computer study randomly assigned 393 heart patients to home prayer groups. Another group of heart patients were not prayed for. Neither the patients themselves or the doctors or nurses who cared for them knew who was in which group.

The prayer groups were made up of people who had "an active Christian life as manifested by daily devotional prayer and active Christian fellowship." They were given only the patient's name, age, and general condition and told to pray for his or her recovery. The un-prayed for group served as the controls.

The results were absolutely astounding. The prayed-for group experienced fewer complications, fewer deaths, and a lessened need for medical interventions. The odds of these improvements among the prayed-for group being due solely to chance was **one in 10,000**, something on the order of being struck by lightning. If the technique being studied had been a new drug or a surgical procedure instead of prayer, it would almost certainly have been heralded as some sort of breakthrough.

I believe in prayer because I've seen the positive results for myself—over and over. I recently met my son, Sean, at the airport, where he was between planes. He was distraught and sick with worry. A television writer, he had spent years creating an original television series, only to learn that it might be given to other writers to develop and he would receive none of the credit. He attempted to get in touch with the series producers but received no return calls.

"What can I do, Mom?" he asked. "I've tried everything I know."

"Sean, there's nothing you can do," I told him. "You've done everything you can, now it is in God's hands." I knew that nothing touches the heart of a loving God more deeply than a mother's prayers for her children. With that in mind, I asked Sean to pray with me, and we went down on our knees right then and there at the airport.

You can't chase happiness. You can only let it catch up to you when you are lost in the giving of yourself.

A few hours later, Sean called me from his home. When he opened his door, he said, the phone was ringing. It was the producer, calling to say he had been trying to reach him, but Sean's phone was out of order. He apologized for what happened and said Sean was right all along. It was Sean's original vision, ideas, and writing that he wanted.

THE FRIENDSHIP FACTOR

Betty, an acquaintance of mine, has a social calendar that looks like an airline timetable. She goes to so many social and professional gatherings that I swear she once signed her own guest book. Yet, she recently confided to me, when a personal disaster struck, she didn't know one person she could call.

I'm not surprised Betty has no friends she can claim as her own. It's not the capacity for intimacy that she lacks, but the time to establish it. The fact is, one cannot have a profound connection with more than a few people. Time prohibits it.

Friendship isn't how many friends you have, but how closely you are connected. Getting close to a few people is more important than being popular enough to receive 300 Christmas cards every year. Like money, your time is finite. You must wisely choose with whom you want to spend it.

A close community, along with the support of friends, helps its members live longer and better lives. Emotional support by itself provides so many health benefits that it's no wonder we instinctively reach out to others. We know what's good for us.

How can you find friends and support in your community? Meet your neighbors. Learn their names and greet them when you meet. Take regular walks. Volunteer at your local church or school. Does the school have a parent/teacher organization? If you work during the week, look into weekend activities and help out. Finding people with common interests is the key here. Does your neighborhood have a local recreation or community center? Ask if your skills can be used in a class or if you can volunteer. Getting involved in life means getting involved with people. Don't be afraid to let them into your life. You'll learn, grow, and benefit greatly. Find people with whom you have common interests. Political parties have auxiliary groups, your local Parent Teacher's Association, neighborhood associations, food banks, church groups—they all need your help.

Here, once again, the law of sowing and reaping applies. If you want something in your life, you must give. If you want respect, give respect. If you want understanding, give understanding and a listening ear. If you want unconditional love, give unconditional love! We rely on the law of sowing and reaping every day when we sit down to eat a healthy meal. No farmer haplessly throws out seed without expecting a harvest. He knows if he continues to tend those seeds in due time they will yield a harvest. Give to others what you want in your own life, and you will receive an abundant harvest. As you plant blessings in other people's lives, God plants blessings in yours. It is this ideology on which I have based my life. Take my word for it, you will reap an abundant harvest. It may not come from the source you expect, but it will come. Cast your bread upon the waters, and it will return one-thousand fold.

In a talk he gave at Washington State University, Warren Buffett, one of the world's richest men, said, "You should hang around the people you admire the most. Then emulate the qualities they have that you most admire. Conversely, look at the qualities you don't like in people and make a point to never duplicate them. My friends enrich my life, making me a better person for having known them."

Look at the people you know who seem the happiest and most satisfied with life. You'll find they are the ones who cherish friendships. Look at them. Discover what makes them good friends and emulate (and appreciate) them.

Nobody I know better epitomizes friendship than my companion and confidante Heide Betz. Even when life's tribulations threaten to make me feel old and ineffective, Heide's support and guidance, integrity and trustworthiness keep me feeling young, confident, vital, and empowered.

When I look in the mirror I see my weaknesses, my faults, and my imperfections. When I see myself in Heide's mirror, I witness my strengths, abilities, and beauty. Heide sees what's best in others and shows it to them brilliantly. Her comments are always sincere, she is quick to repeat any compliment, and she never repeats disparagement.

On my answering machine I once had a message reminding people that "scent always lingers on the hand that gives roses." Heide needs no reminders. She lives this philosophy. My respect for her glows in the light of her confidence.

Following her example, I give my friends freedom. Everyone requires privacy, thus giving them the freedom to work out their problems. Once you say something negative about another person, you lose the option of changing your mind about them.

Why? Because once your confidant hears your complaints, they will understandably make a judgment on your behalf, a judgment not so easily swayed. Beware who you talk to when you have little spats with your significant other. The two of you may resolve the issue later, but your confidant's opinion, because he or she may not be involved in the resolution, will not be so easily changed.

Heide listens but suspends judgment. She artfully leads you through questions that allow you to arrive at your own solutions.

The way to win friends is not by making yourself the focus of attention, but by letting others know you care.

She then acknowledges your conclusions by praising your problem-solving ability. Her every social interchange is done with consideration for others. She is the Michelangelo of personal relationships, creating harmony between people. The example she sets has encouraged the success of her two sons, Michael and Steven.

The same generosity of spirit she offers to her friends, she extends to her successful business as a world-renowned art dealer. Acquiring valuable and rare artwork from around the world, she sells the artifacts to collectors, encouraging them to donate their treasures to museums around the world.

Because I am culturally challenged, Heide has taken me on as a student. I have toured museums and galleries, learning how the beauty of great art enhances life, a concept that is backed by scientific research. Studying and creating art are therapeutic. Like a melodic sonnet or thought-provoking poem, great art stimulates brain cell growth, while at the same time calming the mind.

While Heide has shown me and many of my other treasured friends how to appreciate and celebrate life, my dear friend Evelyn Keen shows me how to appreciate and celebrate my work. As examples of her ambition and entrepreneurialism,

Evelyn shows me that as burdensome as work sometimes gets, it's not a job, it's a calling. It's a privileged anointing worthy of appreciation.

At 76, Evelyn is a titan of enterprise—loving work as if everything depended upon her, praying as if it all depends on God. She uses prayer as a divining rod, finding God's will in every circumstance of her life.

She lives in Pittsburgh, but every time we meet it is as if we have never been apart. Her sense of mission and service keeps her vitally young (she works 12 to 14 hours a day, seven days a week). She has found herself by forgetting herself. As a result, her advice is sought after by all age groups. She is the president of a vitamin distribution company, and she, as I, see her work not as a job, but as a service—not as selling a product, but solving people's problems.

In our business lives we hire financial planners and business managers, but who helps us manage our personal lives? Who helps keep our heart and nervous system strong when life throws us curves? My personal pillar of strength, wisdom, and competence is my friend Nancy Horton. Nancy is the 911 call of my life. For every crisis of my life she has been there for me, preparing to offer sage advice and assistance. Stability, persistence, and excellent judgment are the characteristics I admire and receive from Nancy.

Nobody should have to face crises alone, and with Nancy at my side, I never do. She has such wisdom and clarity of thought that I trust her advice with my every critical decision. Her stalwart assiduousness and dedication are exemplified by her 48-year marriage to her husband, Jack, and the business they have shared throughout their marriage. Nancy and Jack are partners in every sense of the word, not only in their devotion to others, but in their devotion to each other. They start off each day with an early game of tennis, the happiness, harmony, and love in each other fully evident. You can tell that one of their secrets of success is each other.

Research shows that a generosity of spirit and the ability to put others ahead of oneself are factors that contribute to a long and satisfied life.

One of the most amazing acts of generosity, faith, and devotion I've ever witnessed was when Nancy and Jack supported the *Abundant Living* television program hosted by Reverend Kenny Foreman despite the fact that their business had taken a downturn. The Hortons also generously gave financial assistance to help build the Cathedral of Faith church.

I thank God every day that I am able to include Nancy and Jack among my circle of friends. There is no one for whom I hold greater respect or appreciation.

Like recombinant DNA, my friends make up for my deficiencies. My life's greatest blessings are my many friends. If I had a single flower for every one of them, I could walk forever in my garden. My friends are my mentors, my confessors, and my backbones. Their strength and examples keep me strong and inspired. With their support I endure emotional losses, benefit from their advice and examples, and I am more capable of meeting life's challenges head on.

LOVE AND LONGEVITY

As people live longer and healthier, what we think of as old age keeps going up. When the average life expectancy was only 45 a century ago, you were old at 40. In the 1930s, when life expectancy rose to 63, you were pushing old age at 65. Now in the 21st Century, you'll have to be in your 80s or even 90s to be thought of as aged, twice what it was a century ago!

This new view of aging is transforming our concepts of romance, marriage, and family. If you've finished raising your children in your 40s or 50s, you now have, in effect, a second life-time ahead of you.

For many people, this has meant a second, or even third chance at love. More than 50 percent of all marriages now end in divorce, and 80 percent of divorcees remarry. For many people, "Love may be lovelier the second time around." For those, friendship and social and intellectual companionship can make a relationship thrive long after the children have flown the coop.

If sex is good for health, health is even better for sex. In studies of older people with varying degrees of health, half to two-thirds were still sexually active in their 60s, with only 25 percent or fewer after age 75. Those in poor health were most likely to be celibate.

YOUNG LOVE

Elizabeth Taylor and Mary Tyler Moore have tapped into a secret that men have long kept to themselves. Marrying someone younger than yourself can add years to your life. According to researchers women with younger mates live longer.

The longevity advantage can be substantial. In one study, women in their late 50s had one-third the death rate as compared to women in that age group, if they were married to a man one to nine years younger. Women in their 70s who were married to younger men did even better, with a death rate of less than half of their contemporaries. On the other hand, women married to men up to 14 years older than themselves died sooner than expected.

Getting and keeping a younger man may challenge a woman to take better care of herself, which, in itself, may be partly responsible for the increased longevity. Secondly, there is the mind factor. Just thinking of yourself as younger and acting accordingly can be "anti-aging." But there's a seesaw effect that works to the disadvantage of men (although it might seem sweet revenge to any woman who's ever been left for someone younger). There is a tendency for a couple to create a median "age" somewhere between the two of them, with the result that the men become "older" sooner and, as a consequence, die younger.

CHARMS OF AN OLDER WOMAN

If a man wonders why he should choose an older woman, he need only turn to Benjamin Franklin. A great ladies' man, Franklin flirted with almost every woman he met, young or old, pretty or plain. He was following the tradition of dallying with older women as a strategy before he took a wife. And some writers have suggested a rather uncertain and perhaps embarrassing flirtation with a woman 30 years his junior toward the end of his life. However, he preferred older women as companions. In a letter to a friend, he recommended marriage as "the most natural state of man…in which you are most likely to find solid happiness." But if the friend refused to take his counsel, he professed, then in all his "amours" he should prefer older women to young ones, "because they have more knowledge of the world, and their minds are better stores with observations, their conversation is more improving and most lastingly agreeable." Sounds good to me!

Generosity of spirit and the ability to put others ahead of oneself are factors that contribute to a long and satisfied life.

Franklin himself was an impressive role model for aging— swimming great distances in the Thames River in middle age, and becoming increasingly attractive to women as he grew older. He was in his mid 70s when he served as ambassador to France during the American Revolution. Aristocratic young women swarmed all over him at receptions, tousling his thinning hair, sitting on his lap, and whispering in his ear. He opined that older women are "good" women because they've learned that being bad doesn't work.

LOVE CURE-ALL

Scientists call it psychoneuroimmunology. Others call it the power of love. There is no doubt that the mind can release chemicals more potent that any medicine. Consider the following true story, related in the medical journal *Annals of Internal Medicine* (May 15, 1994).

Fifty-five-year-old "Helen" went to see her doctor. He had been treating her for more than five years since her husband had died. She complained of aching joints, low-back pain, shortness of breath, ingrown toenails, and just general fatigue all over her body. An exam and lab tests showed no abnormalities. Helen complained of pain "everywhere." Upon examining her hands, the doctor found them to be very elegant, yet she said they were painful. Helen told her doctor that she played the piano when she was young, but as she grew older she gave it up and this made her sad. The doctor said to come back in six months.

Two months later, Helen returned and upon being examined, the doctor noted there was a sparkle in her eye, her hair was shimmering, and her complexion made her look much younger than 55 years of age. She was radiant, and the doctor noted it was quite a "startling transformation." Helen explained that she had begun to play the piano at parties. To hear the music as well as see the pleasure in people's faces had created great joy in her life. She had also met a man who loved one of her favorite musicians. She had fallen in love and she was no longer fatigued. All of her aches and pains had vanished.

THE BENEFITS OF TOUCH

Sally M. comes from a family in which, she says, "physical demonstrations of affection were like pulling teeth." Then she married into a large Italian family, where hugs and kisses were not only encouraged, they were practically required. "When we went to a family gathering," she told me, "it would take an hour to say 'hello' and another hour to say 'goodbye.' At first I was put off by all this touchy-feely stuff. But when I visited my own family for two weeks last summer, I felt like I was drying up inside. I found I really missed all that touching."

Are you an easy touch? If not, try becoming one. Our sense of touch is the most important of our five senses. Babies won't thrive if they're not touched, and adults don't do much better. We have a biological need for skin contact. It's one of the reasons why social isolation takes such a toll on health and why older people deteriorate rapidly when they're placed into a nursing home.

The sense of touch is linked directly to the nervous system. The skin can be regarded as an exposed portion of the nervous system. More brain tissue is dedicated to receiving signals from the skin than from all the other sensory organs combined. This mind-skin connection can go both ways.

Touch can be used to change behavior, enhance mood, and improve personal relationships. Indeed, it is absolutely essential for optimal development. Stimulation of the skin in a variety of ways, especially from other people, is as beneficial as making the right dietary choices.

Don't be afraid to touch others in a nonsexual manner—a warm handshake, a friendly hand on the shoulder or arm, and, of course, hugs aplenty for family and friends. Touching brings people closer together and it boosts immune function. Try finding ways to literally reach out to others. You can make a point in a conversation by lightly tapping the other person on the knee. Sit close enough to family members to touch when you're watching TV or reading.

And you don't have to be a therapist to massage someone you care about. By taking turns kneading the back and shoulders, you can add relaxation and de-stressing to the benefits of touching.

MAN'S BEST FRIENDS

My longtime friend, and a brilliant and trustworthy attorney, Scott Tips found this essay on the Internet, and since it so beautifully makes the point, I'm including it here. I wish I knew who wrote it.

"Why did God make dogs? I don't think it was accidental, so why do you suppose hounds are around?

Relationships of any kind are a balancing act between intimacy and independence.

"Recently, I watched an elderly woman trying to recover from a stroke. Her brain was damaged, and her arm was weak, so her therapist brought, of all things, a dog to help out. Instead of completing monotonous drills, the elderly patient threw a bright red Frisbee across the room, and the dog bounced over, picked it up, and brought it back, his eyes begging, 'Throw it again, please!' And she did, over and over and over, forgetting that she was actually working quite hard.

"What possessed God to make dogs anyway? Certainly there are exceptions, and certainly people can breed dogs to bring out the worst in them, but in general, there is nothing more selfless, loving, or patient than a dog.

"Mistreat it and it comes back to you anyway. Ignore it and it never gives up hope that you will be its friend again. Make it wait days to go play, and it will still be ready. It offers you friendship and companionship and in return asks only for food, water, and an occasional scratch behind the ears.

"Why would God bother to make such a creature? I suppose that if dogs were like people, they would eventually give up on us...but they never do. A dog's love is almost impossible to destroy, because it's not a love you earn—it's simply a love you are given.

"In other words, dogs love unconditionally. Unconditional love, unending patience, faithfulness to the very end. Do you suppose, just perhaps, that God made dogs to show us a little something about Himself? Do you think maybe 'man's best friend' is really pointing us to the One who is truly our very Best Friend?

"You could learn a lot about God from a dog."

A great believer in dog and cat therapy, I count my shelter-rescued animals among my best friends. My first Great Dane was in dire need of a rescuer. Little did I realize I would be so richly paid back in joy, comfort, a friend, and a muscle relaxer to beat any pharmaceutical. After a stressful day of work, or after being on the road, just to have him there at my side gave me unconditional love, devotion, acceptance, and renewal.

TAKE A CAT TO BED AND CALL ME IN THE MORNING

My life would not be complete without my cats. Anyone who thinks cats are cold and indifferent haven't gotten to know one. When I am away from home, I miss the presence of my feline friends and their soothing purr, which I find calming.

Now I know why. I recently found information that explains why cats purr. A group called the Fauna Communications Research Institute in Hillsborough, North Carolina, conducted some very interesting research focusing on the possible connection between vibrational frequencies and healing (von Muggenthaler,

Elizabeth, "The Felid Purr: A Healing Mechanism?" 2001—Fauna Communications Research Institute, P.O. Box 1126, Hillsborough, NC 27278).

Researchers there questioned the purpose of a cat's purring. I hadn't given it much thought. I'd always been comforted by my cats' purring. Little did I know they weren't just making me happy, they were healing me.

Research discovered that cats purr not only when they are content, but when they are caged, severely injured, or under stress. In their study they recorded the purrs of all types of cats—wild and domestic, in all kinds of situations—households and zoos. When the frequencies of the purrs were analyzed, it was discovered that the dominant frequency for most cats was exactly 25 Hz or 50 Hz—the most effective frequencies for bone growth and repair.

Being able to freely express your feelings to another human being is one of life's great joys.

There's an old saying among veterinarians: "If you put a cat and a bunch of broken bones in the same room, the bones will heal."

We've all heard about a cat's amazing ability to land on its feet when falling from high places. Cats routinely survive and completely recover from falls that would kill most animals. Called high-rise syndrome, there are many reputable studies that document this. In the late 1980s, researchers documented 132 cases of cats that had plummeted an average of 5.5 stories from high-rise apartments. An incredible 90 percent of these cats survived. A third of them did not require any medical treatment at all. The record for survival from heights is 45 stories; however, most cats suffer from falls of seven stories or more and manage to live.

A recent study evaluated the various health problems presented by 31,484 dogs and 15,226 cats to 52 private veterinary clinics around the country. Lameness and spinal disease were among the top problems of dogs, and 2.4 percent were severely arthritic. Kidney and bladder problems were most prominent among cats, and there was no mention of bone, arthritis, or joint problems.

Hip dysplasia, arthritis, and ligament and muscle damage are all common to dogs, but almost nonexistent in cats. Even myeloma, a cancerous tumor in bone marrow, is practically unheard of in cats, yet quite common in dogs. Any vet will tell you how much easier it is to fix a broken bone and how much quicker it heals in a cat compared to a dog.

Researchers at the Ontario Veterinary College in Canada made some very interesting comparisons between dogs and cats regarding their complications from elective surgeries. They found that complications from castration were as much as 20 times higher in dogs than in cats, and the post-operative problems following ovariohysterectomies occurred twice as often in dogs as cats.

As you plant blessings in other people's lives, God plants blessings in yours.

Cats were also found to have quicker recovery times from elective surgeries, large-skin tissue grafts, and breathing problems. Historically, bone cancer is extremely rare in cats, but common in dogs. The list goes on and on.

Purring appears to be a cat's way of treating itself. Just like humans shiver to warm the body, cats purr at specific vibrational frequencies to promote healing in various parts of their bodies. While a cat's purr is commonly 25 Hz or 50 Hz, the range can extend up to 140 Hz. By changing the frequency of their purring, cats fine-tune their healing abilities.

What makes this research exciting is the fact that these frequencies have already been shown to elicit various healing effects in humans. It's not like most studies, where the work is first done in animals and then we have to see if the same phenomenon occurs in humans. The work on cats was conceived based on work already done with humans.

This same idea can probably help explain some of the healing effects associated with mechanical vibrators, massage, classical music, and even laughter. I've seen reports where individuals claim they can stop their migraine headaches by lying down with a purring cat next to their head.

It would seem that the old wives' tale is correct. Cats do have nine lives. Two million old wives can't be wrong. If you want to fill a home, get a cat. They bring us spontaneity, joy, and a truly healing love.

Pets have been shown (even in cold, hard scientific study) to do what any pet owner already knows. In a study of 96 heart disease patients who had been discharged from the hospital, researchers found that having a pet at home was a stronger predictor of survival than either a spouse or family members. Stroking or touching a pet lowers the blood pressure and heart rate. It is the companionable dog with its wagging tail and nuzzling nose, its undying loyalty and nonjudgmental, unconditional love that protects its master from the stresses of life.

Pets are an incredible blessing. I know from experience. My dog and cats bring me joy, love, and happiness. As the stress of my many responsibilities lowers my shoulders, I see my animals play, cuddle up to me, and look at me with adoring eyes and my heart is lifted. There is little greater joy than to escape into the life and love of pets.

The life experiences that enhance the quality of our lives also carry our challenges and bring hardships and sometimes devastating losses. When we are able to overcome them, we become stronger and more capable. While writing this book, I lost my beloved husband. I lived for him. What sustained me was what I refer to as the three "Fs"—faith, friends, and family. They watered the roots of my soul and healed me. Never underestimate the power and strength of close relationships.

Achieving social security is about extending yourself socially, taking chances, and looking for love. As you sow life's blessings into the lives of others, be assured that God will reciprocate. Honor your friends by giving them space, encouraging them to talk, expressing yourself, taking responsibility for your words, and letting them into your life. Arming yourself with a shield of friendship will be your first line of defense against the adversities, afflictions, and anguish that we have and will encounter and which typically negatively impact human longevity. Relationships replenish the spirit and help us maintain a youthful mindset. We need to be loved, and more importantly, we need to be needed.

Why do some people look younger than their years? Why are some afflicted with arthritis at 40, while others live pain-free into their 70s? How can you protect yourself against the ravages of time and live longer, healthier? The tools for arming your second line of defense are contained in the next chapter, "Your Department of Defense."

CHAPTER FOUR

YOUR DEPARTMENT OF DEFENSE

Strengthening Your Body Against Aging

ld age is a series of challenges, all of which can be overcome. As each challenge is met, you are rewarded with renewed confidence, self-esteem, and an enhanced quality of life. You can win major victories! Preventing and/or prevailing in these battles and prolonging life, health, and beauty requires that we give our body the best defense possible.

WHAT DO WE DREAD THE MOST ABOUT AGING?—arthritis and osteoporosis crippling our bones and joints; wrinkled skin and thin, gray hair, heart disease, debilitating strokes, slow death from disease—cancer? Prevent these pathologies from first occurring, and you can live in good health into your 80s, 90s, and beyond.

Aging is an accumulation of natural processes—not a combination of degenerative diseases. Such diseases are not inevitable. To grow old does not mean to grow sick.

The information and recommendations contained in this chapter and throughout this book will provide you all the ammunition you need to maintain a strong and disease-free body throughout your long and active life.

COLOR ME HEALTHY

Think of the rainbow hues of various foods as a "nutritional flag" of good health. Many foods derive their color from chemical compounds that have anti-aging benefits. For instance, carrots and cantaloupe are colored yellow by the antioxidant beta carotene, and blueberries are tinted by the heart-helping pigment, anthocyanin.

Aging is an accumulation of natural processes—not a combination of degenerative diseases.

Heap your plate with a full palette of colors, and it will nourish your body as well as please your eyes. The following is a color chart along with the corresponding foods and benefits.

• **Blue and Purple.** Blueberries, grapes, blackberries, cranberries, cherries, and raspberries enhance blood circulation and protect the heart. Raspberries and strawberries neutralize carcinogens in the intestines. Raisins, currants, and prunes prevent iron-deficiency anemia, fight cancer, and stimulate immunity. (These are also high in stress-fighting B vitamins.)

• **White.** Potatoes, mushrooms, bananas, and beans (white on inside) inhibit the formation of cancer-causing compounds. Onions and garlic inhibit enzymes that activate carcinogenic chemicals. Fish and seafood protect the heart. (The color rule with fish is the darker, the better, since bluefish, salmon, and other dark-hued fish contain the most omega-3.)

• **Brown.** Wheat germ, oatmeal, nuts, and brown rice contain vitamin E, a major antioxidant that fights cancer, heart disease, and aging. These foods are also rich in fiber, B-vitamins, and iron.

• **Red.** Tomatoes, pink grapefruit, and watermelon contain lycopene, a cancer-preventive antioxidant. They are also high in vitamin C, the immune-boosting antioxidant that helps prevent the formation of cancer-causing nitrosamine in the stomach.

• **Yellow-orange.** Carrots, sweet potatoes, cantaloupe, apricots, papaya, and mango contain beta carotene, a precursor of vitamin A that has been shown to prevent cancer in many studies.

• **Yellow.** Corn and yellow peppers contain beta carotene and vitamin C. Tumeric, a spice used in curry, and yellow mustard inhibit cancer formation in animals. Mustard also contains isothiocyanates, which stimulate cancer-protective enzymes.

• **Green.** All green vegetables contain chlorophyll, the same chemical that makes plants green and binds to cancerous chemicals in the stomach and prevents absorption. These include leafy greens, kale, beets, turnip greens, broccoli, green peppers, and kiwi. Green herbs such as basil, mint, and parsley contain anti-cancer antioxidants.

Grapes and their seeds are full of anti-aging nutrients. Purple and red grapes—and the wine and juice made from them—contain anti-inflammatory, anti-cancer, and anti-aging nutrients credited with repairing connective tissue, protecting the liver from toxins, reducing pain and swelling of varicose veins, and revitalizing aging skin. Grapes contain the antioxidant anthocyanin and resveratrol, a powerful phytochemical. Resveratrol protects the heart and blood vessels by decreasing stickiness of blood platelets, boosting good (HDL) cholesterol and blocking the bad effects of bad cholesterol. Its anti-inflammatory effect can also protect against Alzheimer's and other brain-related illnesses. Anti-aging studies have shown people who drink one glass of (red) wine a day live longer and have fewer age-related diseases. For teetotalers, purple grape juice offers the same benefits.

SUPPLEMENTAL NUTRITION TO HELP THINGS ALONG

Even if you believe in three square meals a day, you cannot possibly get all the nutrients you need from the food you consume.

Here are six reasons why even the best food is not enough to give your immune system all it needs to ward off disease:

1. Heavy farming exhausts our soils and depletes them of nutrients. Today's farming techniques create sterilized soils by not allowing the land, from which the plant mines its minerals, to rest each seventh year in order to remineralize.

2. Stressors, such as injury, illness, and difficult situations, exhaust the body's store of nutrients.

3. We can't possibly eat the amount of food it takes to nutritionally reverse the debilitating effect of time.

4. The 2.2 billion pounds of pesticides poured onto our produce, coupled with the chemicals we use and are exposed to every day, mean our bodies need more vitamins and minerals to combat their effects.

Heap your plate with a full palette of colors, and it will nourish your body as well as please your eyes.

5. Processed food: zero calories means no nutrients whatsoever; hidden transfats (hydrogenated anything) and chemicals, dyes, and preservatives. White bread and refined sugar don't give you vitamins and minerals. They *require* them to be digested. If a food doesn't feed your body, don't eat it.

6. Food sensitivities and allergies interfere with digestion, the absorption of nutrients, and repeatedly rally the body's defenses until the adrenals are exhausted. In addition, most of the time you aren't even aware of it!

Aging is many things, but not exclusively a loss of cells. Rather, a major contributor to the aging process is damage to every cell in the body by what science prefers to call "free radicals." Free radicals are technically known as reactive oxygen species (ROS), in essence meaning excess toxic breakdown products of oxygen.

Increasing evidence suggests a role for free radicals, or ROS, in all disease processes.

There are naturally occurring ROS and, due to today's proliferation of industrialized food processing and chemicals, an abundance of man-made ROS in the environment. When the body's enzymatic ability to cope with excess oxygen toxic byproducts is overcome by the sheer numbers of these byproducts, disease occurs.

Cell membranes are largely made up fats (lipids). "Inclusion structure" mitochondria in each cell produce 95 percent of the cell's energy in the form of oxygen. Oxygen escaping in the "unpaired" form of so-called free radicals, or ROS, burns everything it touches—like the sparks in a barbecue pit. When free radicals puncture and damage the cell membrane, the process is called lipid peroxidation.

At this stage in biochemical research there is sufficient evidence to link oxygen free radicals (ROS) with such aging problems as cataracts, circulation blockages, Parkinson's, Lou Gehrig's disease, arthritis, and wrinkles, just to name a few.

Anything that increases oxygen in the cells increases free radicals. This includes illness, inflammation, prolonged stress, and exposure to ultraviolet radiation. When we sunburn, free radicals have used up antioxidants in the skin, causing the burn. Forty-five minutes of direct sun on the face uses up all the skin's vitamin C reserves.

There is enough research and evidence to conclude that antioxidants are our first line of defense. What are the main antioxidant vitamins? Simply think ACE—vitamins A, C, and E.

Vitamin A protects the thymus from the effects of chemicals, poisons, and anything else that stresses the immune system. Without adequate A the skin becomes rough, dry, and ages prematurely. It also assists in healing wounds, night vision, preventing infection and ulcers. One cup of carrot juice contains 24,750 Individual Units of vitamin A.

People who take vitamin C live longer, a lot longer. A study found that daily supplements of vitamin C given to people starting in middle age or older increased their life-span by six years for men and by one year for women. Humans need to take vitamin C because our bodies don't produce it. When animals are given drugs, including alcohol, nicotine, and caffeine, their bodies go into high gear, producing large amounts of vitamin C to detoxify the drugs. We can't do this. What we can do is slowly increase vitamin C up to bowel tolerance. For most healthy people, this means three to six grams (3,000-6,000 milligrams) a day. When we are ill, our tolerance—and thus our body's need—may increase to 20 to 30 or more grams per day.

Taking vitamin E is like having a private army defend you against all potential enemies. In the past five years, much evidence has accumulated regarding its effectiveness with respect to so many different conditions that even conventional doctors (who once ignored the vitamin) are sitting up and taking notice. At a meeting of the American College of Cardiology, nearly two-thirds of the cardiologists in attendance revealed that they took supplements of vitamin E and/or other antioxidants.

Vitamin E has now been shown to have beneficial effects in preventing heart disease and cancer, enhancing the immune, endocrine, and nervous systems, protecting against environmental pollution, promoting wound healing and healthier skin, and reducing inflammation. According to a report in *The American Journal of Clinical Nutrition*, vitamin E, in doses of 800 Individual Units per day over a month, enhanced important measures of immune function in a group of 32 healthy women and men over the age of 60 when compared with untreated controls.

Any discussion of antioxidants should include lipoic acid, an antioxidant critical to the vitamin A-C-E network. Supplemental lipoic acid—specifically alpha lipoic acid—facilitates metabolic pathways and helps convert food into energy. It is used in Europe to prevent some of the side effects of diabetes and oxidative stress.

Using it on patients with mushroom poisoning, Dr. Burton

Berkson found it elicited immediate relief and reversed the toxic effects on their livers. It has also been found helpful for heart problems and brain injuries.

The studies are so compelling that I recommend alpha lipoic acid for any chronic degenerative disorder involving tissue breakdown.

Other awesome antioxidants are selenium, which works with vitamin E, coenzyme Q10, a valuable preventive for heart problems, and the amino acids glutathione and methionine.

STAYING IN CIRCULATION

Can you say "vasodilators"? They are nutrients that give your arteries greater smoothness and flexibility, allowing them to push blood through more quickly and easily. They can help whenever a lack of blood flow (circulation) becomes a problem. This can include arterial blockages, heart problems, painful muscles, memory loss, Reynaud's, or numbness in the extremities.

Nutrients credited with being vasodilators are vitamin E, vitamin C, vitamins B12 and B3, the mineral magnesium, and the amino acid arginine. L-arginine is commonly used to treat peripheral vascular disease. The herb ginkgo biloba helps memory loss because it increases blood flow to the brain.

To grow old does not mean to grow sick.

Vitamin E makes the blood cell more malleable, so that the eight-micron blood cell can squeeze through the four-micron capillary/blood vessel. It also aids the heart and other vital organs in getting a healthy blood supply.

The Bible says life is in the blood. Magnesium is prescribed for heart problems and protects the brain and heart from toxins and inflammation from any source. In one study, 75 percent of people were found to be deficient in magnesium. Magnesium and the vitamins B12 and B3 are the great vasodilators, including the aforementioned new kid on the block, ginkgo biloba.

Blood flow can also be restricted by blood clots, induced when the body undergoes trauma, whether from accident or surgery. Any surgery that involves the veins and arteries, especially heart surgery, includes the risk of artery-clogging blood clots. Typically, surgical patients are given a blood thinner, usually heparin, to prevent this from happening. Doctors and nurses must be trained in the use of heparin because of a common side effect. It's so common they gave it a name: heparin-induced thrombocytopenia (HIT). As many as 30 percent of surgical patients experience this side effect, which, if it goes unrecognized, can result in life- or limb-threatening circulation blockages from blood clots. How ironic, indeed, that a drug given to prevent something causes the very thing it is trying to eliminate. Even more ironic is that the medical establishment, instead of looking at alternatives to heparin, is attempting to develop medications to counter its side effect. Scandalous, indeed, is medicine's refusal to acknowledge an alternative to heparin that has been shown to be safer and more effective.

Chondroitin sulfate, commonly used for arthritis, is related to, but distinct from heparin. Heparin must be given intravenously. Chondroitin sulfate is absorbed in the stomach, so it can be taken orally. The body retains it twice as long as heparin, and it is absorbed more thoroughly. Clinical studies have shown that it works better than heparin in preventing blood clots and without the dangerous side effects.

MINERALLY RICH LIVING

Minerals are the building blocks of enzymes. When there is a deficiency in minerals, the enzymes that catalyze all the body functions cannot work properly. Lacking minerals, the metabolic and digestive enzymes can't break food down properly so it can be absorbed by the body.

The availability of minerals to the body is more important than the total amount of minerals you take in. Swedish researchers found that the harder the water in terms of the minerals it contains (calcium, magnesium, zinc, copper, boron, and the trace constituents), the lower the death rate from cardiovascular disease and stroke. Their studies revealed that people who drink water highest in minerals have 41 percent fewer heart deaths and 14 percent fewer strokes.

Although water is a relatively small source of minerals, the difference could be due to the fact that the minerals are in solution, allowing for the most rapid and effective means of absorption by the body. Putting trace minerals into liquid form ensures the greatest bioavailability.

Antioxidants are our first line of defense against aging. Simply think ACE—vitamins A, C, and E.

Zinc is a component of more than 200 enzymes and is needed for more enzymatic reactions than any other mineral in the body. Many older people are marginally deficient in zinc, which means that their enzymes do not function at peak efficiency and their immune system is compromised. A deficiency of zinc can lead to increased infections, poor wound healing, a decreased sense of taste or smell, and skin disorders.

The thymus, the traffic cop of the immune system, requires zinc in order to manufacture and secrete thymic hormones and for the protection of the thymus against cellular damage.

Adult-onset diabetes is on the increase, and one reason is the lack of chromium in today's diet. Chromium is a major regulator of insulin, and its deficiency in the body can be a leading factor in heart disease and diabetes. Adequate levels of chromium, as well as vanadium and the B vitamin biotin, not only protect the body against these two diseases but increase immune resistance to germ-caused disease and infections. And it may slow the aging process. Studies have shown that low chromium levels can accelerate aging, while optimum levels keep aging at bay.

Imagine driving your car without checking the oil and replacing it when it runs low. At some point you would run it into the ground, perhaps ruining it forever. Many people do something similar to their bodies when they let it run low on magnesium. This mineral is as important to performance of your body as oil is to your car's engine. It propels about 80 percent of the body's enzyme reactions. It is vital for your heart, blood pressure, energy level, and overall cellular function, yet most of us do not get the magnesium we need on a regular basis.

THE CALCIUM/MAGNESIUM CONNECTION

The process of aging is what researchers and doctors call calcinosis, meaning calcium is pulled from the bones and deposited into soft tissue, settling in your arteries, joints, and skin, causing arthritis and the pale, hard, wrinkled look of aging. When you are born, your cells are 95 percent magnesium and five percent calcium. Under a microscope they are translucent. As you age, your cells degrade to 95 percent calcium and five percent magnesium.

Relieving stress is important because stress increases the body's need for vitamins and minerals. Long-term stress requires long-term nutritional support. Over time, stress can also cause calcium to be pulled from the bones and deposited in the tissues. When this happens, the calcium can crystallize, causing cross linkages. Other aging-associated problems then develop: arthritis, wrinkles, blockages in the arteries, cataracts, and shriveled sex glands.

Calcinosis occurs because of a very common deficiency of magnesium. This deficiency can start as early as the teenage years. A magnesium deficiency is very serious, and, based on the available research, is probably the number one cause of death from disease. It even plays a role in cancer.

For years doctors and health care experts have been advising us to get enough calcium. So, you dutifully drink your milk, eat your cheese, and take calcium supplements. But something is still wrong because many of us still experience osteoporosis, heart disease, fibromyalgia, hypertension, cancer, arteriosclerosis, and wrinkles. What is missing, and what has been shown in studies to make a tremendous difference, is the addition of magnesium.

All the minerals work in concert. Look around at the way God orders nature. He never creates a mineral in isolation, always in concert, like a symphony. Magnesium needs the other minerals to perform to its maximum potential.

Magnesium should be taken in a mineral formula, at least two to one with calcium. Foods high in magnesium—and missing from the typical diet—are whole wheat, nuts, dark green vegetables, and molasses. One cup of pumpkin seeds has 738 mgs. of magnesium. I mix pumpkin seeds with dried cranberries, which contain flavonoids. They taste terrific, are a hardy snack, and are a harmonious color blend.

DHEA—THE ANTI-AGING HORMONE

Dehydroepiandrosterone (DHEA) may be a candidate for a spelling bee tie-breaker, but it's as hard to ignore as a thousand-pound gorilla. DHEA is produced in the adrenal glands and is plentiful in youth. But by the time you're 80, you have only 10-20 percent of the amount you produced in your second decade of life. Many gerontologists believe that DHEA may be the best biomarker for aging and longevity.

Adequate levels of DHEA mean you are less likely to develop a large number of age-associated diseases and conditions, including atherosclerosis, cancer, diabetes, and a decline in mental function leading to dementia, Alzheimer's, and Parkinson's disease. It can help protect against a variety of other ailments, including autoimmune diseases, osteoporosis, viral and bacterial infections, including AIDS, memory loss, learning disability, emotional problems, depression, and stress. There are also indications that DHEA may extend the life-span.

Supplementing your diet with vitamins and minerals will go a long way in combating the effects of aging.

I get my DHEA from a progesterone cream. It increases bone density, alleviates symptoms of menopause, and prevents age-related weight and water gain, all while helping to protect me from cancer, heart disease, and osteoporosis.

DHEA also nourishes the brain and helps alleviate the effects of stress, memory loss, and inability to reason. A recent study of men in nursing homes found that their levels of independent functioning were directly related to their DHEA levels. It has been determined that DHEA helps heal wounds and improve bone density and muscle strength. When it comes to supplementing with DHEA, take it easy. The secret is to start low and slow. No more than 25 milligrams should be taken supplementally, as it can cause temporary hair loss and changes in hair follicles. For optimum benefit, use it topically in cream form so it can slowly be absorbed into the body and assimilate naturally.

CELL THERAPY

While not yet approved in the U.S.—where at this writing it seems to be in the process of co-optation under such terms as "xenotransplantation" and "fetal cell transplantation therapy"—live cell (or cell) therapy has long been used in Europe to treat a variety of illnesses.

It does not replace a good diet, supplements, and exercise, but if you've been neglecting your body or you suffer from a degenerative disorder that threatens your life, cell therapy can give you the opportunity to level the playing field. What you do from there will help determine how well and how long you live.

Modern explanations of this approach, based on ancient documents as well as 20th Century research, have determined that the injection of suspensions of birth-related tissues, often from the endocrine system, works as a kind of "organ transplant," making cells "act younger"—just as a young puppy will encourage his tired old canine companion to imitate his friskier behavior.

Cell therapy has the multiple ability to help regenerate or heal damaged organs and tissues and, perhaps more importantly, to balance the entire hormonal or endocrine system, which in effect influences every other system.

Greatly advanced in the modern era by Paul Niehans, M.D., a noted Swiss specialist in the field of gland and organ transplants, cell therapy is used to stimulate healing, counteract the effects of aging, and treat a variety of degenerative diseases such as arthritis, Parkinson's, atherosclerosis, and cancer. I have seen it transform Down's Syndrome children.

Progress in cell therapy in the U.S. has largely been stymied because of the conflict over the experimental use of aborted human fetuses in medical research. Notwithstanding, and as most live cell proponents point out, birth-related human tissue is not only absolutely not needed as a source of cells, but, at a time of universal panic over spreading human viruses, is positively counter-indicated. In most venues, cell therapy involves the use of cellular suspensions from the embryonic, fetal, or placental tissues of animals. While the debate over human tissue rages on, stem cells from animals are nearly identical and often provide the same benefits.

The basic theory behind cell therapy was best stated by Paracelsus, a 16th-century physician who wrote: "Heart heals the heart, lung heals lung, spleen heals spleen; like cures like." Paracelsus and many other early physicians believed that the best way to treat illness was to use living tissue to rebuild and revitalize ailing or aging tissue.

Modern orthodox medicine lost sight of this method, so it now uses chemicals to interrupt or override living processes. While chemicals and drugs work only until they are broken down by the body's metabolic processes, cell therapy has a long-term effect because it stimulates the body's own healing and revitalizing powers, often successfully revitalizing and extending youth. Cell therapists see their patients' skin tone and complexion improve, an increase in vitality, their youthful optimism and energy return, and various other infirmities of aging much improve.

In Germany, more than 5,000 German physicians regularly administer cell therapy injections. A great proportion of those injections are funded by the West German social security system. Since the mid 1950s, several million patients the world over have received cell therapy injections, including such celebrities as Bernard Baruch, Marlene Dietrich, Gloria Swanson, Sophia Loren, Henry Kissinger, and at least one pope, to name just a few.

While considered a controversial treatment (in the United States), be aware that cell therapy is practiced world-wide on a daily basis. Blood transfusions and the transfusion of various other blood components, such as red blood cells, white blood cells, and blood platelets, are accepted forms of cell therapy. Less commonly, implants of the cells of the thymus have been utilized—essentially without as much as a wink of the eye of medical authorities.

Much of the controversy in the U.S. surrounds the belief that human fetal tissue must be used. However, it is completely unnecessary because, as previously mentioned, animal cells are identical at the fetal level. Cells from neonatal pigs have the same beneficial effect and are just as compatible.

Cell therapy, which involves three sets of injections, has been found to be beneficial in treating the following maladies: general loss of vitality; physical and mental exhaustion; convalescence after illness; premature aging; signs of deterioration of the brain, heart, kidneys, lungs, liver, skin, and digestive organs; lack of drive and declining mental efficiency; weakness of the immune system; arthritis and other degenerative diseases of the connective tissue; underfunction of the endocrine glands; disturbances of menopause; Parkinsonism; Alzheimer's; autoimmune diseases; chronic pain; and atherosclerosis of the brain and heart and peripheral circulation; organ repair; and even cancer.

Rodrigo Rodriguez, M.D., offers cell therapy at the International Bio Care Hospital & Medical Center (IBC) in Tijuana, Mexico. He explains, "Our cells are programmed to die. These new neonatal animal cells are programmed to live."

A graduate of George Washington University who pioneered in nuclear medicine for 20 years, Dr. Rodriguez interned in Toronto, then chose to return to his homeland because it was only there that he was free to use up-to-date healing techniques otherwise not sanctioned by the U.S. FDA.

Bad news travels the fastest, and many Mexican clinics do not earn good reputations. However, I have observed firsthand Dr. Rodriguez' work at the Center, and it exceeds American standards for sanitation, comfort, and service. The IBC staff are sent to the Ritz Carlton in Hawaii so that they can learn what constitutes first-class service. IBC offers state-of-the-art treatments for age-related problems (including weight loss), full-spectrum lighting, delicious all-organic food from an award-winning kitchen, and no synthetic fabrics or detergents touch your skin, as they use only cotton sheets, towels, and gowns washed in organic soaps.

Ginkgo improves mental capacity, mental alertness, sociability, and mood, and can reverse memory loss.

I have also observed the healing of the incurable with cell therapy and wellness programs using a variety of therapies. I saw a man with Parkinson's put into remission, and a beautiful 33-year-old Italian woman, Paola Cassolari, cured of cancer. Paola had been told by numerous cancer experts that she had two weeks to two months to live. When the cancer that started in her breast moved to her spinal column, she began a desperate search that ended with a successful program of nutritional supplements and treatments at the International Bio Care Center. She returned home, healthy and whole.

For more information contact Rodrigo Rodriguez, M.D., at the International Bio Care Hospital & Medical Center in Tijuana, Mexico, www.ibchospital.com or call 1-800-785-0490.

You should note that the extraordinary healing I saw at IBC took place by incorporating more than cell therapy. If you've lived for 50 years, you may have been taking supplements for the past ten years, perhaps low-dose vitamins for the past 35 years. We are the first generation to discover the benefits, but we're running behind younger people who have been taking supplements most or all of their lives. We need a little help. Cell therapy can help get your health back, but supplements, a proper diet, and exercise must always be included in order to ensure a long and healthy life.

EARMARKED HERBALS

Only recently have scientists zeroed in on what Chinese healers have known for thousands of years—ginkgo biloba is useful for treating many of aging's symptoms.

Ginkgo biloba circulates blood quickly through the vessels, helping to avoid clots and blockages. Because of this, it has a remarkable revitalizing effect on the brain. Ginkgo improves mental capacity, mental alertness, sociability, and mood, and can reverse memory loss. Ginkgo leaf extracts are the leading prescription medicines in Germany and France. In the U.S., ginkgo biloba, at a standard 24 percent flavonoid concentration, is available as a nutritional supplement.

For most people, the recommended dosage is 120 mg daily. It takes time for natural botanicals such as ginkgo to build up to the concentration needed to realize the full benefit—anywhere from several days to six weeks. There are few, if any, adverse side effects associated with its use.

For additional anti-aging benefits, look for a formula that includes DHA, which is an omega-3 triglyceride derived from fish oils. DHA enhances brain function, helps thin blood, reduces inflammation, lowers blood pressure, loosens stools, and lowers cholesterol.

The history of garlic for medicinal purposes stretches back 5,000 years and across many continents. In ancient times, the Babylonians, Egyptians, Phoenicians, Vikings, Chinese, Greeks, Romans, and Hindus frequently used garlic to cure intestinal disorders, flatulence, worms, respiratory infections, skin diseases, wounds, symptoms of aging, and other ailments.

Extensive research has revealed that garlic is an impressive antioxidant and detoxifier. Constituents in garlic not only scavenge free radicals, but they also increase one of the body's major antioxidants—glutathione.

Kyolic Aged Garlic extract was used successfully as part of a nutritional program for the Russian children of Chernobyl. The aging process removes the irritants, toxicity, and odor from raw garlic.

DON'T SWEAT IT

For those of you who really hate heavy, stressful workouts, I have good news. Strenuous exercise is not the best idea. It increases free radical activity, stresses the joints, and as you breathe heavily, you take in more pollutants faster. Science is now saying it is *moderate* exercise that prevents illness, increases health, and promotes mental vitality.

Exercise is the unanimously uncontested age reverser. It is credited with reversing heart disease, diabetes, hypertension, osteoporosis, depression, and mental problems. It increases circulation, strength, bone mass, immune system function, and mental vitality.

An important, scientifically proven benefit to exercise is that it promotes *initiative thinking*—creativity and motivation. Many of the world's most successful writers took long walks before writing. Scientists have since learned that when the body is exercised, the brain becomes more active. Before you make that difficult decision, take that important test, or start writing that best-selling novel, take a long walk. You'll be amazed at how easy and fast the ideas and solutions come to you.

Most of us want to lose weight. If you want to lose weight *and* gain strength, do it with weight-bearing exercise. Three one-hour workouts at low intensity actually burn off fat better than six 30-minute sessions at high intensity.

You may not be 86 yet, but it's comforting to know that even at that late hour, you can still reverse the effects of having been a couch potato. My workout buddy Edna Markus lifts weights and rides a stationary bicycle. She can push 50 pounds off her chest and lift 30 pounds with both legs. Edna is 86 years old. "Before I started," she said, "I found everything hard—shopping, cooking, walking. I felt wobbly; I held on to a wall when I walked. Now I walk down the center of hallways. I feel wonderful." Edna's family was prepared to place her into long-term nursing care. Instead, they enrolled her in a special seniors weight-training program three times a week. Now she lives independently in her senior apartment complex surrounded by friends young and old who seek her out because she makes them feel good about themselves.

Of course, what constitutes moderate exercise is different for everyone. To me, moderate exercise is a game of tennis, racquetball, or golf. What is important, no matter what your age, is tailoring your exercise to your fitness level and enjoying what you do.

According to my personal trainer, Chris Mullen, these are the symptoms of overstressing yourself with exercise: insomnia, muscle soreness, frequent injury, and a compulsion to exercise even when you are sick. Less is more. Chris recommends waiting at least 72 hours after muscle fatigue so healing can take place.

Moderate exercise prevents illness, increases health, and promotes mental vitality. Exercise is the unanimously uncontested age reverser.

I work out regularly at the Power House Gym in Redwood City, California, owned by Rob and Stephanie Soufla. I am energized not only by the exercise regimen Chris puts me through, but also by the facility's sparkling and sun-filled environment. It has huge windows that let in the sunlight. Sunlight is a nutrient and programs your body for sleep. I do a noon aerobics class and find that without it, I don't sleep as well. Try to include at least 15 minutes of sunlight with your exercise, and you'll find you sleep better.

A MERRY HEART DOETH GOOD LIKE A MEDICINE

There is an anatomy of joy, says William Fry, Jr., M.D., a Stanford University psychiatrist and pioneer in laughter research. The muscles of the abdomen, neck, and shoulders rapidly tighten and relax, the heart speeds up, the blood pressure rises, breathing becomes spasmodic and deeper. It happens whenever we let ourselves go in dancing, running, and jumping for the fun of it. It also occurs when we laugh so hard our whole body is convulsed with mirth. "One hundred laughs is equal to ten minutes of rowing," says Dr. Fry. "Sustained hilarity is among the more agreeable form of aerobics."

The most astonishing evidence of laughter's power comes from a 1997 study of 48 heart attack patients. Half watched comedic television shows for 30 minutes every day, and the other half watched dramas. After a year, ten patients in the drama control group had suffered repeat heart attacks, compared with only two in the same group that watched comedy shows.

THE IMPORTANCE OF HYGIENE

Henry Ford didn't know it, but he started a revolution in longevity. By inventing the assembly line, he made mass production of cars, which led to dump trucks that could cart our garbage away all over the country. The improvement in sanitation was the main reason that we added another 25 years of life to the average life-span in this century.

The nutritional and exercise practices that I have outlined in this chapter are only two sides of a triangle that bring you within striking distance of the potential life-span of 120 years. The third side is personal hygiene. That's another 50 years just for washing your hands properly. A proper hand-washing technique includes scrubbing under the fingernails and using warm water and plenty of soap.

The word *hygiene* is derived from Hygeia, the ancient Greek goddess of health. It was the cornerstone of healing then, and it has not changed to this day.

Consider this: Less than 150 years ago, the unwashed hands of doctors were responsible for the deaths of one in four women in childbirth. Today, only one in 100,000 women die in childbirth, and surgery is infinitely safer because of simple handwashing, which remains by far the most effective—and neglected—means of preventing the spread of infection.

The most common infections, including colds, are spread not through the air, but by the hands, specifically under the fingernails, to the nose, eyes, and mouth. Mucus is the stick board for viruses and bacteria. You can reduce your chances of getting these infections by 90 percent if you regularly follow this procedure: (1) Dig your fingernails into the soap to clean out the area where the germs are nesting and then wash your hands. (2) Immerse your face in a basin of warm water containing a small amount of the solution. Pretend you're an underwater swimmer and open your eyes in the water in order to flush the front of the nasal passageways and eyes. (3) Finally, blow your nose into a clean tissue and repeat the procedure until there is no more mucus in your nasal passage. In this way, you close the doors to germs.

Your soap should kill germs by boosting the skin's own defenses. The skin is perfectly capable of keeping itself clean. Scientific studies have shown that the skin has its own defense system. For myself, I have formulated an antibacterial soap made of natural herbs and botanicals, such as hawthorne extract, a bioflavonoid that has anti-cancer properties, increases circulation, and is used in heart medicine. Another ingredient is comfrey, which contains the healing agent allantoin. Comfrey has wound-healing properties and is used to treat leg ulcers. No matter how often I use it, it never causes dryness and heals red scaled skin on my hands and body.

For your arsenal against disease, infections, and maladies, cleanliness is an important line of defense. Get in the habit of washing your hands and bathing daily, and you'll find yourself on the go while others you know are laid up in bed.

GETTING WHAT YOU NEED
FROM WHAT YOU EAT

We may be star stuff, but as we age our stars grow progressively dim. We lose the minerals that keep our bodies young and vital. The reason we lose these minerals even if we eat healthy whole foods is because most older people have a deficiency of stomach (hydrochloric) acid. This deficiency prevents the absorption of minerals into the bloodstream because the food cannot be properly broken down without it.

Many people are surprised to learn that a major problem of aging is **lack** of stomach acid and the accompanying enzymes, as opposed to excess stomach acid. Commercials on television are always telling us that when the foods we like don't like us back, we should take antacids. The clear implication is that heartburn, gas, bloating, and abdominal discomfort are due to too much acid, not too little. In fact, the way that nature ages us and slowly ushers us out this world is to cut back on the flow of hydrochloric acid and the accompanying enzymes in the stomach. This deficiency causes food to stay in the stomach too long, allowing it to rot and putrefy, creating gas, acids, and toxins.

While orthodox medicine continues to focus on excess stomach acid, a number of studies and authorities clearly refute this. Researchers have determined that by 60 years of age, 60 percent of people have a significant decline in hydrochloric acid. Others have found even higher percentages of stomach acid deficiency in the older population.

According to *Dr. Braly's Food Allergy and Nutrition Revolution*, "Eighty percent or more of food-allergy sufferers have different degrees of hypochlorhydria (a lack of hydrochloric acid in the stomach)...which leads to the pancreas's inability to secrete enough digestive enzymes and alkalinizing bicarbonates."

The standard test for measuring the amount of hydrochloric acid present in the stomach is called a Heidelberg test. It involves swallowing a little capsule that reads out to a computer, indicating when it is in the stomach or small intestine and the locality's degree of acidity and alkalinity. It is one of the most accurate tests used in medicine today. If you want to locate a doctor who offers the Heidelberg test, contact my office at 1-800-445-HEAL or www.mksalaman.com.

Malabsorption, the inability to absorb nutrients, can also be caused by stress, illness, and certain pharmaceutical drugs. Anything that alters the natural chemistry of the intestines and stomach, especially antacids, can prevent vitamins and minerals from being broken down and absorbed.

Minerals are especially difficult to absorb. Getting calcium from antacids doesn't work, because without stomach acid, calcium cannot be absorbed. You can't absorb vitamins without the proper amounts of minerals. Intestinal problems can keep B vitamins, essential to mental health, from being absorbed. Pernicious anemia, a deficiency of vitamin B12, is associated with depression, as is irritable bowel syndrome. If you suffer from depression and have problems with your small intestine, consider the possibility they are linked.

At the risk of sounding like your mother, always chew your food! Those who do not masticate, nature castigates. Twenty to 30 bites is a good "rule of tongue." Chewing properly helps prepare your food for digestion.

Take supplemental digestive enzymes. Enzymes are essential for digestion and aren't always available from food. Don't eat on the run. Play soft, slow music. The feel of a soft napkin, the glow of candles, all prepare the stomach for digestion like instruments contributing to a concert. Mozart wrote table music, and all these years later science has proven its validity. As always, remember to take your minerals in solution to maximize their absorption.

THE INFLAMMATION ANSWER

I recently attended an anti-aging conference in Monaco. There I was able to converse with many eminent doctors in the field. One particularly compelling testimony came from a laboratory biochemist from Milan by the name of Marc R. Rossellini. Through a massive ten-year, $26 million study on aging, he discovered something that only a few of us knew: the number one epidemic and killer is not heart disease or cancer, or the next ten leading diseases. The number one epidemic and killer is chronic inflammation/autoimmunity (CIA)—the process the body uses to defend itself from harm. Trauma from an injury causes the body to first react (autoimmunity), then attempt to heal and protect itself by collecting fluid (inflammation) in the tissues surrounding the injury.

Good nutrition, adequate exercise, and personal hygiene will bring you within striking distance of the potential life-span of 120 years.

Medical experts estimate total CIA-related diseases currently affect approximately 190 million Americans, or over 69 percent of the total population. CIA is the single systemic factor in over 90 percent of the 2.4 million deaths caused by the ten most common diseases.

Rossellini states that chronic inflammation of epithelial cells (skin and internal tissue) is a systemic factor for 80 to 90 percent of all diagnosed cancers, heart disease, and organ disease.

ENZYMES FOR DIGESTION AND DISEASE PREVENTION

Rossellini's information was nothing new to me. I'd learned long ago that chronic inflammation—swelling that causes pain—can be treated with enzymes. Enzymes have been used clinically to treat the inflammation and edema that typically follow oral surgery.

I take two different digestive enzymes formulas. One is designed to break down in the stomach and release its enzymes so my food is thoroughly digested and I receive maximum nutrition from it.

In the other, the product that prevents chronic inflammation, the tablets are coated so the enzymes are released in the bloodstream in lieu of being digested in the stomach. This mimics the benefits of enzyme-packed food like fresh fruits and vegetables, preventing the chronic inflammation that promotes illness and disease. Enzymes break up debris in the injured area, decrease the swelling, and stimulate the body's own natural enzymatic processes, without causing the immune system to be suppressed (as occurs when cortisone is used to fight inflammation). Enzymes also keep trophoblast cells in check, preventing their overgrowth and mutation, which contributes to uterine fibroids, heart disease, endometriosis, fibrocystic breasts, ovarian tumors, and cancer.

In cancer prevention, blood circulating enzymes de-shield the cancer cell, allowing the body's natural defense system to recognize it as a foreign invader and destroy it. Blood circulating enzymes also work for fibrocystic disease because they digest necrotic tissue (toric tissue in scientific terms).

Advocates of enzymes for sports injuries indicate that, although the type and extent of the injuries vary so much, the anti-inflammatory effects are confirmed again and again. Two of the sports physicians who were assigned to care for the German Olympic teams carried out a controlled investigation and obtained "good" to "very good" success rates in 82 percent of the athletes under their care. They did so with the relatively low dose of only two or three tablets three times a day.

I take about 12 enzyme tablets a day on an empty stomach. I've already identified and eliminated foods to which I am allergic. For me, it is most effective to take them before I go to bed (at least one hour after eating). They reduce inflammation (which is the cause of all pain) and keep my eyes from being puffy in the morning. Because of this reduction in swelling, a delightful side effect is that they also help reduce wrinkles.

AVOID ANTIBIOTICS

Life-threatening, invasive fungal infections have risen dramatically in the past two decades. The main reason is increasing use of antibiotics. Every time antibiotics are used, the bacteria they are supposed to kill mutate to defend themselves. As a result, many of conventional medicine's arsenal of antibiotics have become ineffective against some infections.

In poorer areas of the world where antibiotics are not used, fungal infections are extremely rare. But in industrialized countries, such as our own, they are becoming a significant cause of illness and death.

The fungus Candida, which can cause serious and debilitating disease, has become the fourth most commonly isolated pathogen in blood cultures. Those who are most at risk are individuals whose immune systems have been weakened by organ transplants, cancer therapy, use of broad-spectrum antibiotics, and HIV.

ALTERNATIVES TO ANTIBIOTICS

Long before drug companies started manufacturing synthetic antibiotics, people were using the ones found in nature.

All types of infection respond to vitamin A, especially those that affect body tissues, like pneumonia, skin infections, and ear infections.

Over 50 years ago scientists first discovered vitamin A's value in treating and preventing colds and flu. In areas of the world where vitamin A deficiencies are common, a higher percentage of children are blind and suffer from chronic infections.

In an amazing discovery, it was determined that vitamin C is helpful in the continuing battle against bacteria that otherwise have developed an immunity to antibiotics. Antibiotics are not the most desirable way to fight infection, but they continue to be used. Today, medicine is in a quandary because so many of the bacteria we are fighting have become immune to antibiotics. Rather than using stronger antibiotics, physicians should consider using stronger doses of vitamin C.

A recent Harvard study found vitamin C may reduce bacterial resistance to antibiotic therapy. In their laboratories researchers exposed strains of staph bacteria to ascorbic acid for six hours. In four of the six strains, the bacteria showed less resistance. The researchers found that the doses of antibiotics could be reduced by 50 to 75 percent after resistant strains of bacteria were exposed to vitamin C.

They also found that previously ineffective doses of penicillin and tetracycline showed increased inhibitory effects on resistant bacteria, and in some instances the vitamin C even killed 23 to 93 percent of the initial bacteria population. This was a very exciting discovery. With vitamin C, not only are old antibiotics once again useful, but you don't have to take as large a dose.

When you target vitamin C as a supplement, choose a formula that includes bioflavonoids and green tea. Bioflavonoids are potent anti-inflammatories. Among other therapeutic benefits, they reduce swelling, boost the immune system, and enhance the healing properties of vitamin C.

Researchers conducted several well-designed studies that revealed when vitamin C was combined with bioflavonoids, the levels of vitamin C in the blood were higher and remained higher longer than with vitamin C supplements that did not contain the bioflavonoids. Green tea contains the bioflavonoid catechin, which strengthens the tiny capillaries of the body and polyphenols, natural chemicals that fight cancer.

MY SINUS FLUSH

A large and grateful segment of the population was saved from Chicago's 1918 influenza epidemic that killed 8,500 Chicago residents. Allopathic doctors helpless to save themselves and their patients flocked to osteopaths who successfully used the sinus flush to treat patients. For this reason alone there still exists an osteopathic hospital in Chicago. I tell people to add this remedy to the infection chapter in my book *All Your Health Questions Answered Naturally*.

First, fill a hot water bottle with warm water. Add a teaspoon of salt to turn it into a saline solution. Put the plastic tube in it and the water regulator, which is provided, on the tube. Lower your head parallel with the sink with your mouth open, breathing rapidly. This closes the glottis, preventing water from dripping down the throat.

Cut the tube at an angle and gently insert it into your nostril, slowly letting the water go into the sinus cavity, flushing out all the filth that has been living right behind your nose and eyes.

Do this three times a day. You'll feel completely revitalized and refreshed. You'll notice the swelling around your eyes disappear as the air circulates through your newly cleaned, clear passages. It feels wonderful. Infections from bronchitis to pneumonia start from the sinuses and drip down the back of the throat. As the viral and bacteria-laden mucus is trapped, it works its mischief on your bronchial tubes and lungs, causing throat and lung infections. The sinus flush prevents this from occurring.

In the interest of understanding why sinus problems become chronic, you should understand catarrh. Catarrh is the term used to describe the response of the mucus membranes to infection and allergies. It means inflammation of the mucus membranes, causing excess secretions. The underlying cause may be allergies, but when too much mucus is secreted (as bacteria grows in the mucus), the result is painful infection. The body responds to two primary commands: cleanse waste and build cells.

A runny nose is your body's attempt to cleanse waste. But when the mucus of a runny nose goes from thin clear to thick yellow or green, it is not able to cleanse waste anymore and has become a storehouse of bacteria. Get rid of the mucus and you rid yourself of the bacteria, infection, and irritation.

The beneficial effects of nasal irrigation for chronic sinusitis are obvious to anyone with this condition who has irrigated regularly. However, it was not until a group of physicians in Madrid, Spain, performed a study on allergy sufferers that the benefits of irrigation for allergies was documented. They found that irrigating the nose with saline three times a day during the grass pollen season (May to July) significantly reduced the allergic response to grass. In addition, it allowed the sinus membranes to heal.

Pollutants inhaled during our daily breathing is like rubbing delicate sinus tissues with sandpaper. They need the added protection and strengthening of vitamin A, beta carotene, and vitamin C with flavonoids. I take them daily in a formula made from natural sources.

In closing this chapter, I want to reiterate that the tools and means to stay healthy longer are available to you. Supplemental nutrition is the key to arming your immune system so that illnesses, diseases, and common maladies do not get the best of you, and you optimize your defenses. With this information in hand, you *will* live longer, **better**.

5

"I wish above all things
that thou mayest prosper
and be in health,
even as thy soul prospereth."

3 JOHN 1:2

CHAPTER FIVE

BATTLES THAT HELP YOU WIN THE WAR

Overcoming the Diseases of Aging

ost Don't Want to Live to Age 100, Poll Finds."
This was a headline that didn't surprise me.
When confronted with the possibility of living to age 100, a telephone survey
of 2,032 adults found that 63 percent preferred not to. Declining health
was the most common reason for rejecting longevity.

NOW, ASK YOURSELF. Would you want to live to 100? What if you knew you could live to be 100, be disease free, and retain vibrant good health? What if you knew you could live without cancer, osteoporosis, Alzheimer's, heart disease, cataracts, or arthritis? What if you could feel vitally healthy all the time? Your answer would probably be "yes," and if you read on, I will tell you how to help prevent and/or conquer these maladies.

DIETARY HELP FOR MENOPAUSE

If there's one issue with plenty of misinformation and hysteria regarding middle age, it's menopause. The fact is, the symptoms of menopause—hot flashes, night sweats, insomnia, and irritability—among others, can be prevented! How else can you explain why some women go through the change unscathed, while others cry desperately for help? The answer is the adrenals. The adrenal glands form the baby-making hormones estrogen and progesterone. As the child-bearing years are left behind, the adrenals make less of these hormones, and fluctuations occur. The condition of the adrenal glands seems to determine how short-lived these symptoms are or whether they occur at all.

Would you want to live to 100? What if you knew you could live to be 100, be disease free, and retain vibrant good health? Your answer would probably be "yes."

Have you ever experienced a hot flash of embarrassment or a "rush" of adrenaline when on a roller coaster? You know how when you're very angry or frightened your blood rushes to your head and you feel almost dizzy? These are your adrenals' responses to stress. It is these same stress responses that cause menopausal symptoms. As the adrenals stop making estrogen, the body responds to the stress.

Exercise is essential in any program of stress or menopause relief. The reason the adrenals excrete more hormones when we are under stress is to make us physically ready to fight or run. Every once in a while you will read about somebody under stress performing an incredible feat of strength—lifting a car to save someone, for example. If that person had not taken action when his body told him to, he would have suffered. Stress and menopause both require a physical outlet to "work off" excess hormones so they don't turn inward and damage the body.

Hot flashes. Every menopausal woman gets them, right? Wrong! If they are such an inevitable symptom of menopause, why then do women in some cultures not experience them? Although Americans consider hot flashes nearly universal symptoms of menopause, investigation does not bear this out.

Cross-cultural studies have found that Mayan women say they don't experience hot flashes; Greek women experience hot flashes but shrug them off as trivial; and while a small proportion of Japanese women report hot flashes, they are far more likely to complain of headaches and stiff shoulders. Japanese women don't even have a word for hot flashes. What makes the difference is their diet. The cultures that don't experience high incidences of hot flashes typically eat foods high in phytoestrogens—foods that naturally contain estrogen—that can help normalize hormone levels.

Legumes—soybeans, peas, beans, and certain roots—are isoflavonoids, which act as a non-steroidal estrogen. Soybeans, a fabulous cancer fighter, are eaten in great quantities in Japan and China, and are the reason researchers believe these countries have low rates of breast cancer. Tofu, soybean curd, is not as bad tasting as it sounds. It has the unique ability to absorb the flavors it is cooked in. Other oestrogenic foods include apples, carrots, yams, green beans, peas, potatoes, red beans, brown rice, whole wheat, rye, and sesame seeds.

Now that you know about soy, look for my favorite soy snack, "Maximum Living Nutrition Bites." It is packaged as chewy nuggets and comes in three flavors: chocolate, vanilla nut, and peanut butter. The soy protein in these tasty snacks contains many other vital nutrients, including fat-reducing enzymes, fiber, nitrogen, and amino acids.

There is another reason why these foods stabilize estrogen needs: they are high in dietary fiber. Fiber is capable of altering the way various estrogen hormones are metabolized. In one study, women showed significant reductions in a form of estrogen (estrone) after two months on a high fiber diet. Estrone is associated with hormonal problems. Fiber helps the liver metabolize estrogens so levels can be normalized and balanced according to need. The best source of fiber is hyssop. When choosing fiber supplements, look for a product that contains hyssop, psyllium, oat bran, and acidophilus for a healthy bowel. Psalms 51 says, "Cleanse me with hyssop that I might be clean."

THE DANGEROUS SIDE EFFECTS OF HORMONE REPLACEMENT THERAPY

On July 9, 2002, The National Institutes of Health announced that it had halted a major study, stating that the long-term use of estrogen and progestin significantly increases the chances of invasive breast cancer, blood clots, and heart attacks. The study was to continue until 2005.

The study was stopped when they realized that not only was the hormone therapy unlikely to benefit the heart, but that after just a year-long use of estrogen and progestin the women in the study were threatened by an increased risk of heart attack (by 29 percent), breast cancer (by 26 percent), and stroke (by 41 percent).

Hormone replacement therapy (HRT) also may worsen menopausal symptoms and increase the risk of endometrial and breast cancers, fibrocystic breast syndrome, edema, uterine fibroids, and bone weakness.

Currently, six million American women take this potentially lethal hormone combination, under the long-standing assumptions that it was a safe and effective way to combat the symptoms of aging and menopause. There is no joy for me in telling women "I told you so" when the NIH finally validates what I have been saying for 38 years. For years the pharmaceutical industry has embraced its billion-dollar business based on research skewed to show what they wanted us to believe.

It is a well-known scientific fact that women who take hormone replacement therapy have healthier lifestyles than the general population. They get regular exercise, take nutritional supplements, eat more fruits and vegetables, drink water instead of soft drinks, etc. This bias alone easily explains a decrease in breast cancer deaths.

Contributing factors skewed the research. As the "researchers" looked at one group who used HRT and another who did not, they discovered that the subjects who were not on HRT did not take good care of their health. They didn't exercise, take nutritional supplements, eat healthy foods, etc. These were factors, which the researchers did not take into account, that invalidated the study. All factors in a study must be consistent and known. The study should have been placebo-controlled with both healthy and unhealthy subjects evaluated. Half get a placebo and the other half get HRT, with neither aware of which they are getting.

In addition, the studies only looked at women who have ever used hormones, not taking in account how long they were on them. The women could have taken hormones for one month or 10 years. There is agreement that it is both current use and duration of use that increase breast cancer incidence and deaths. The most recent report from the Nurses' Health Study showed that the mortality advantage from taking HRT was partially counteracted after 10 years of use because of the increase in deaths from breast cancer. What will happen after 20 or 30 years?

The fundamental problem with using HRT for prevention is the notion that a drug with any potential risk should be used to prevent a future disease that may or may not occur. As the most recent Nurses' Health Study pointed out, women who live a healthy lifestyle—nonsmoking, not obese, normal cholesterol, normal blood pressure—have no significant advantage from taking HRT. Lifestyle changes are an option that should not be so easily dismissed.

IDENTIFYING AND REVERSING ESTROGEN DOMINANCE

Hormones link together in your body to be effective. If one

chain is missing, all the rest down the chain are missing. As if it weren't bad enough that as we get older our progesterone stores diminish, synthetic hormones also cause us to become progesterone deficient. It's not a lack of estrogen that causes deadly diseases and symptoms of PMS and menopause. It's too much estrogen—estrogen dominance.

Hormone replacement therapy makes the problem worse because synthetic hormones, especially progestin, fool the body into thinking it doesn't need to make progesterone. The drug most commonly used for hormone replacement therapy, Premarin, is made from pregnant mares' urine. It's got all the right hormones, if you usually dine on hay. Pharmaceutical companies don't use naturally derived hormones because if they didn't tinker with its molecules, creating a mismatch to the human body, they couldn't make it an expensive, patentable drug.

The American Journal of Epidemiology reported on a study in which premenopausal women with low progesterone levels were found to have 5.4 times the risk of developing breast cancer and experienced a 10-fold increase in deaths from all malignant tumors when compared to women with normal progesterone levels.

In the U.S. it is common for women's production of progesterone to fall to near zero, often six to eight years before actual menopause. It is commonly believed that estrogen levels also plummet as a woman nears menopause. This is a fallacy. Low premenopausal progesterone levels increase estrogen to a point where it dominates the system. This explains why the most common age for breast cancer is five years before menopause, and why so many women in their early 50s are being diagnosed with the disease.

Even men have estrogen dominance because of our daily exposure to 2.2 billion pounds of estrogen-mimicking pesticides and the synthetic estrogens used to fatten cattle, pigs, and chickens, and to increase milk production.

Fortunately, there is much we can do to overcome estrogen dominance. Two natural hormones, melatonin and DHEA (dehydroepiandrosterone), have connections to the adrenals, and those ties have proven to be advantageous to menopausal women and older men. DHEA is an androgen, one of the hormones reduced during menopause, and studies have shown that melatonin's effect on estrogen could quite possibly reduce the risk of breast cancer.

I use a natural, non-synthetic multi-vitamin formula that is high in B complex vitamins from organic vegetable sprouts (the most potent form for nutrients possible), with extra choline and inositol added. It helps the liver break down estrogen into estriol, a non-carcinogenic form of the hormone (estradiol is the carcinogenic form). B vitamins also can reduce many of the symptoms of premenstrual syndrome.

Certain foods can help with the estrogen/breast cancer link. Three kinds of flavonoids—deltanoids, retinoids, and terpenoids—have the same properties as Tamoxifen, a pharmaceutical drug (with major side effects) that keeps breast cells from absorbing estrogen. Terpenoids are found in abundance in rosemary and citrus oil (the oil you squeeze out of the pores of citrus fruits); retinoids are precursors of vitamin A and are found in orange fruits and vegetables; and deltanoids are found in egg yolks.

In a report published in *Chicago Medicine*, the bioflavonoid hesperidin, found in citrus fruit rind, was a more effective treatment than sub-therapeutic doses of estrogen for menopausal symptoms.

NATURAL PROGESTERONE CREAM FOR ESTROGEN DOMINANCE

I recently participated in a physicians' panel with John R. Lee, M.D., a renowned expert on menopause. We spent many hours discussing solutions to the problem, and I was fascinated by his success with natural progesterone cream to counter estrogen dominance and its menopausal effects.

The doctor found that among those patients who were using the progesterone cream, serial lumbar DPA tests showed an increase in bone density, as opposed to an anticipated delayed loss. He notes one patient had a pathological arm fracture at 72, and after using natural progesterone cream, at 84 her bone density increased 40 percent and she had no fractures.

It should be obvious that healthy and long living means healthy eating. You are what you ingest, digest, and expect, as well as what you have inherited.

Encouraged, Dr. Lee started using progesterone cream on patients already on estrogen and realized similar results: their bones got much stronger. His patients reported other benefits: increased alertness and energy; relief of breast fibrocysts and painful breast swelling; recovery from mild hypothyroidism; decreased need for aspirin or NSAIDs (non-steroidal anti-inflammatory drugs), and, most unexpected of all, a return of normal libido—and with no side effects.

In over 20 years of practice, Dr. Lee has found that progesterone alleviates menopausal symptoms like hot flashes, facial hair, male pattern baldness, vaginal dryness, and loss of libido without the dangerous side effects related to the use of synthetic estrogen.

Progesterone is a natural compound, and it cannot be patented by drug companies. It is not the same as progestins, which are synthetic progesterone. Progestins have side effects that include breast cancer, facial hair growth, depression, cardiovascular disease, liver disorders, and other associated problems. Synthetic progesterone makes the body forget to make progesterone, resulting in estrogen dominance.

Natural progesterone, manufactured in laboratories from

wild yams and soybeans, easily converts natural progesterone into the identical molecule made by the body. Natural progesterone cream can be used by both men and women for prevention of bone loss and osteoporosis. Natural progesterone has no feminizing effects.

Be aware, however, that yam-derived natural progesterone is not the same as "yam extracts" that are sold in health food stores. The body cannot convert yam extracts into progesterone.

When taken orally, progesterone is not absorbed into the body. However, it is particularly well absorbed by the skin. In postmenopausal women, progesterone cream may be used two to three weeks of the month and then discontinued until the next month. In perimenopausal women it is used from about day 12 to day 26 of the menstrual cycle, because the body may become insensitive to the effects. It is recommended that it be discontinued for at least five to seven days each month.

Women on estrogen should reduce their estrogen dose in half when starting progesterone. Many will be able to eliminate or reduce their estrogen intake in the next several months.

For those on Provera who want to use natural progesterone, taper off the progestin gradually. You can do this by cutting the progestin dose in half for the first month as the progesterone cream is added. Then cut in half again the second month, taking it every other day if necessary. By the third month the progestin can be safely discontinued. When considering a new therapy, it's best to consult with a nutritionally educated physician.

For a list of physicians versed in nutritional therapy, call the National Health Federation at 626-357-2181. They charge a nominal fee of $10. This money is well spent for the oldest health freedom organization in the world. The NHF is the reason you are free today to buy nutrients over the counter.

OSTEOPOROSIS

When you get aches and pains, it's because your body is trying to tell you something. As you get older, your body becomes more talkative. The signs are noticeable long before the diagnosis: general weakness, hip and back pain, muscle tenderness and cramping, periodontal disease, decreased height, stooped posture, and the beginnings of a "dowager's hump." Older patients may suffer a severe vertebral compression fracture by merely stepping off a curb, or fracture a wrist in a slight fall. Finally, and most mysteriously, some patients, for no apparent reason, fall with a broken hip. The actual reason: the hip joint deteriorated to the point that it could no longer support the bones above.

Often it isn't until one of these bad breaks occur that osteoporosis is diagnosed for what it is, and not dismissed as fatigue, poor posture, or a nagging backache. By the time it is diagnosed, as much as 50 percent of the bones' spongy mass has been lost.

Everyone knows that calcium strengthen bones. That's why we drink milk, right? Wrong! You've seen billboards pronouncing "everybody needs milk?" They should change it to read: Everybody needs...sesame seeds, kelp, spinach, chard, brewer's yeast, sardines, carob, caviar, soybeans, almonds, torula yeast, parsley, Brazil nuts, watercress, salmon, chickpeas, egg yolk, and beans. These are the many varieties of foods that are high in calcium—and low in fat and synthetic hormones.

Only 25 percent of women taking calcium are in fact preventing osteoporosis. While calcium supplements were found to increase bone mass in these women, it had no impact on the other 75 percent. Why? Because there are many other factors that can prevent calcium from being absorbed by the bones. The balance of nutrient intake is very important in ensuring calcium is absorbed in the body. Too much of one nutrient, or not enough of another could mean the difference between strong bones and broken bones.

A recent study found a link between excessive intake of calcium supplementation and clogged arteries. Researchers using powerful new imaging technology scanned the arteries of 39 young dialysis patients and found nearly 90 percent of those in their 20s had serious coronary artery calcification. Calcium deposits had crystallized in their arteries, a form of cardiovascular disease expected in 60- or 70-year-olds, although virtually unheard of in young people. The study, published in the *New England Journal of Medicine*, found patients with the stiffest arteries ingested 6,000 milligrams of calcium a day, twice as much as kidney patients whose arteries weren't calcified.

One reason for brittle bones may be a shortage of vitamin D. Among elderly patients with hip fractures, 10 to 20 percent have impaired bone mineralization because of vitamin D deficiency. The same deficiency is also responsible for something called osteomalacia, or bone softening. Because it causes bone weakness, it is similar to rickets in children.

A major source of vitamin D is sunlight on the skin. However, with the risks and warnings associated with ultraviolet rays, many people avoid or sharply reduce their exposure to the sun. The problem is, they don't make it up by eating enough vitamin D-rich foods.

Probably the best source of vitamin D is cod liver oil. Before you say "ugh" and make a face, you should know that it now comes in many tasty flavors, like strawberry, cherry, mint, and citrus.

The best foods for vitamin D are sardines, salmon, tuna, egg yolk, sunflower seeds, liver, cheese, cottage cheese, and bee pollen.

Other factors that keep calcium from being absorbed are too much protein, especially in meat. One long-term study found that with as little as 75 grams of daily protein—less than three quarters of what the average meat-eating American consumes—

more calcium is lost in the urine than is absorbed by the body.

To get your daily allowance of complete protein combine whole grains with legumes. Other protein plant food combinations are nuts and seeds with legumes, and nuts and seeds with dark green leafy vegetables. Consider a green salad with kidney beans and sunflower seeds. There you have it: a good source of protein and lots of other essential nutrients! Beats a steak any day, and you'll save money!

The true fruition of our mature years is wisdom, insight, and a deeper, fuller, richer, more satisfying mental life.

Too much phosphorus also causes a loss of calcium. Yet, not enough may have the same effect. For optimal absorption, the ratio of calcium to phosphorus must be one to one. Most American diets contain a one to four ratio of calcium to phosphorus. This is because commonly eaten foods such as meat and potatoes are high in phosphorus.

So-called soft drinks could be hard on your bones. A Harvard University study of nearly 5,400 female college grads, ages 21 to 80, revealed that for ex-varsity athletes over 40—a time when estrogen levels and bone mass decline—drinking nonalcoholic carbonated beverages more than doubled the risk of bone fractures. It also took the fizz out of exercise's bone-strengthening benefits.

The high amount of phosphorus in soft drinks depletes calcium (as the body tries to balance out the ratio of phosphorus to calcium). So, if you value your bones, swear off the "soft" stuff.

As an alternative, concentrate on the foods that have close to a one to one ratio. They are: radishes, Brie cheese, apples, pears, boysenberries, cranberries, pineapple, watermelon, Swiss chard, eggplant, summer squash, and green beans. High-calcium, low phosphorus foods include: kale, sesame seeds, maple syrup, and seaweed.

One of the best kept secrets in biochemistry is the fact that vitamin K, well-known for its contribution to blood-clotting, is a star performer in assuring strong, solid, healthy bones. It is also required to synthesize osteocalcin, a protein found uniquely and in large amounts in bone.

Many people become deficient in vitamin K because they don't eat enough vegetables or because they take antibiotics. Foods high in vitamin K include cheddar cheese, Camembert cheese, Brussels sprouts, soy lecithin, alfalfa, oats, spinach, soybeans, cauliflower, cabbage, broccoli, liver, potatoes, and bran.

Magnesium, a neglected nutrient in American diets—especially in women—contributes to the making of solid, enduring bones by changing vitamin D to its active form and by activating an enzyme that helps create new calcium crystals in the bone. Dietary surveys have shown that 80 to 85 percent of American women consume less than the RDA for this mineral. Foods rich in magnesium include kelp, blackstrap molasses, sunflower seeds, wheat germ, almonds, soybeans, Brazil nuts, bone meal, pistachios, soy lecithin, hazelnuts, pecans, oats, walnuts, brown rice, chard, spinach, barley, coconut, salmon, and corn.

Very important, and not emphasized enough, is the danger of taking calcium without magnesium. Magnesium is the traffic cop that tells calcium where to go. Without it, calcium leaves the bones, where it's needed most, and infiltrates the soft tissues, crystallizing and causing a plethora of problems, from arteriosclerosis to severe and early wrinkling of the skin. Science terms this syndrome calcinosis.

Focus on foods that contain potassium, calcium, and magnesium. They include: wheat germ, sunflower seeds, soybeans, almonds, brazil nuts, pistachios, and pecans. Each of these foods can be added to salads, cereal, and snack foods. Conveniently, they have a pretty decent shelf life as well.

Another unsung hero is **manganese**, which is a must for

synthesizing connective tissue, structural material in both carti-
lage and bone, and for assuring that needed minerals will be
retained in our bones. Foods high in this mineral include sea-
weeds, tea leaves, cloves, ginger, buckwheat, oats, hazelnuts,
chestnuts, wheat, pecans, barley, Brazil nuts, sunflower seeds,
watercress, peas, beans, almonds, turnip greens, walnuts, brown
rice, peanuts, honey, coconut, pineapple, and parsley.

Until recently, even leading biochemists had no idea that the
trace mineral **boron** could be useful in human nutrition, let
alone in the maintenance of bone health and integrity. One particular experiment rocked them like an earthquake. When three
milligrams of boron were added to a typical daily diet of postmenopausal women, the amount of calcium they excreted in
urine dropped by 44 percent. At the same time, the blood concentration of the most biologically active form of estrogen rose
sharply—to the same level as experienced by women receiving
estrogen therapy.

How does boron work this wonder? At this point, biochemists
have offered only an educated guess. However, when boron joins
certain organic chemicals, it appears to facilitate the synthesis of
the most usable form of estrogen. Foods rich in boron include
beans, peas, lentils, nuts, pears, leafy vegetables, soy meal, prunes,
raisins, almonds, peanuts, hazelnuts, dates, and honey.

Silica is another lesser-known mineral, found where calcium
is deposited in sites of growing bone. It appears to strengthen the
connective tissue matrix by crosslinking collagen strands. Chicks
fed a silica-deficient diet developed gross abnormalities of the skull
and had unusually thin leg bones. Best sources of silica are the
fiber portion of brown rice, bell peppers, leafy green vegetables,
and the herb horsetail. As an alternative, look for a liquid mineral formula derived from natural sources that contains silica,
potassium, phosphorus, and magnesium, as well as calcium.

Minerals in solution are more easily and completely absorbed into the body.

Exercise, especially weight bearing, is essential for avoiding osteoporosis. I do aerobics to stay slim, walk to stay healthy, and lift weights to keep my bones strong. Obese people may have heavy hearts, but their bones are typically thick and strong from carrying all that weight. Remember, you have to pick yourself up and start moving in order to realize any benefit.

ENLARGED PROSTATE

Contrary to conventional wisdom, prostate problems need not be an inevitable part of aging. Yet, if you look at the statistics for enlargement of this life-giving male gland, you may arrive at that conclusion. By age 50, twenty percent of American men have benign prostatic hyperplasia (BPH—a fancy term for enlargement); by 70, half the population will be affected; and by 80, over 80 percent. Just as breast cancer is rare in countries where plates are filled with vegetables and whole grains rather than meat and dairy products, so too prostate problems are uncommon in non-Western cultures.

That's the bad news. The good news is that in most cases prostate problems can be prevented through a healthy lifestyle that features a low-fat, nutrient-rich diet.

The Center for Complementary and Alternative Medicine at the National Institutes of Health in Bethesda, Maryland, is charged with evaluating alternatives to conventional therapies. Grants paid for by the Center include double-blind studies that show saw palmetto (Seronoa repens) to be as effective as conventional drugs in treating an enlarged prostate. The herbal extract is nontoxic, and the cost is approximately 60 percent less than Proscar.

European physicians have long known about the benefits of

saw palmetto and utilized it for BPH. Doctors in France prescribe Permixon for their BPH patients. Permixon is made by Pierre Fabre laboratories in Paris and consists of only one ingredient: saw palmetto. In Spain, physicians prescribe Sereprostat for prostate problems—again, 100 percent saw palmetto.

Other herbals, available in health food, vitamin and drug stores, have been found to be helpful not only for prostate enlargement, but for sexual prowess as well. Ginseng has been used for centuries by the Chinese culture to increase energy and libido. It works by increasing circulation and blood flow, thereby boosting the immune system, washing out toxins, and putting nutrients where they belong.

Equisetum arvense is commonly known as horsetail, and it can help men maintain their "stallion" status. It is high in the mineral silica, noted for its help in reducing the inflammation of prostatitis (a prostate infection) or prostate enlargement. Horsetail is often combined with Hydrangea arborescens, commonly known as hydrangea, which is also highly effective in the treatment of inflamed or enlarged prostate glands.

An enlarged prostate may lead to prostate cancer. Researchers at Johns Hopkins University and at Roswell Park Memorial Institute found men with an enlarged prostate were four times more likely to develop cancer than those with normal prostates.

For a healthy prostate, pass on the pizza and red meat. Researchers are finding that a diet high in fat is linked to prostate cancer. It is estimated that with a reduction in dietary fat, 81 percent of prostate cancers are potentially preventable. My award-winning book *Nutrition: The Cancer Answer* has numerous succulent lipid-lowering recipes and more on prostate cancer.

One study discovered that people who ate liberal amounts of vegetables containing beta carotene (carrots, sweet potatoes, yams, cantaloupe, apricots, spinach, squash, and leafy green vegetables) had a lower risk of prostate cancer. Vegetarians who, for the most part, eat less fat have a lower incidence of cancer of the prostate than men with high fat intake. A vegetarian diet lowers circulating testosterone levels and a meat-eating diet raises them. Prostate cancer grows on testosterone and slows when testosterone is lowered. A study of Japanese men conducted in 1977 noted that the marked increase in mortality from prostate cancer paralleled the increase in fat intake in the Japanese diet since 1950.

There is good fat and bad fat. The bad fat is **trans** fat contained in margarine and hydrogenated processed foods, as well as saturated fat in a primarily meat diet. The good fats—the ones that help take bad fats out of the body—are the oils: olive, walnut, flaxseed, and borage oil supplements. Raw oil goes rancid quickly when left unrefrigerated. Dip flaxseed bread in extra virgin olive oil for a special treat.

In summary, if you suffer from the common malady of an enlarged prostrate or BPH, supplement with an herbal supplement containing saw palmetto, pygeum, and horsetail, pass on high fat foods like pizza and red meat, and instead eat vegetables and seed oils. You should find yourself a lot more comfortable with your prostate, and the rest of your body will also realize some benefit.

ALZHEIMER'S

A generation ago, many people were resigned to slowly losing their mental powers as they grew older. Senility, dementia, loss of memory and mental acuity, and even depression were thought to be an inevitable accompaniment of old age. We now know these symptoms are signs of sickness, not age, and that the true fruition of our mature years is wisdom, insight, and a deeper, fuller, richer, more satisfying mental life.

But what about those diseases of the mind? They are the

most dreaded aspect of growing old. Perhaps no other disease strikes such terror into the hearts of older people than Alzheimer's. It's a death sentence for the mind, as though a thief came in the night, entered your brain, and began removing your most precious possessions—the very memories that make you who you are. Although conventional medicine has failed miserably in making a dent in this disease, alternative therapies are enjoying considerable success.

Two environmental toxins, aluminum and mercury poisoning, particularly from silver amalgam dental fillings, have been linked to Alzheimer's. If you have a mouthful of silver amalgam fillings, find a dentist versed in the newest plastic fillings (called composites) to replace them. Many insurance companies cover them. They are the same color as your teeth, are more durable, and contain no mercury to poison your brain.

Certain nutritional deficiencies have also been tentatively tied to Alzheimer's. These are: folic acid, niacin (B3), thiamine (B1), B6 (pyridoxine), B2 (riboflavin), vitamin C, vitamin D, vitamin E, magnesium, selenium, zinc, and tryptophan.

Nutritional supplements can be highly beneficial for Alzheimer's patients. Studies in Japan have shown that daily supplements of coenzyme Q10, vitamin B6, and vitamin B12 returned some Alzheimer's-diagnosed patients to "normal" mental capacity. Another study found that evening primrose oil, zinc, and selenium improved alertness, mood, and mental ability in Alzheimer's patients. I use borage oil instead of primrose oil. It has 26 percent more of the healing agent gamma linoleic acid and is one-fourth the price.

Nutritional supplements are also important for patients with Alzheimer-like symptoms who are actually suffering from cardiovascular problems. Niacin can help to improve circulation, large doses of vitamins C and E lower cholesterol, and because it is estimated that 40 percent of all senile patients are deficient in this B vitamin, folic acid is important.

A balanced mineral intake is essential to both prevent and treat mineral deficiencies that may play a role in Alzheimer's disease. Once again, for optimal absorption, choose a mineral formula in solution.

Several studies have shown that ginkgo biloba may be useful in treating Alzheimer's. In a six-month trial, it was found to enhance memory retention in Alzheimer's patients.

Antioxidants are super-duper nutrients that seek out and destroy the free radicals that ravage and destroy our skin, joints, tissues, organs, and bones.

While no one knows exactly what causes Alzheimer's, there are intriguing indications that it could be an allergic disorder, perhaps a form of chemical poisoning. There certainly are enough chemicals in our environment these days, and nobody disputes the fact that silver amalgam fillings contain mercury, or that the amounts of aluminum in our food and medicines, in some instances, far exceed safe levels.

The warnings are not taken seriously because not everyone develops Alzheimer's. Then again, not everyone gets hay fever.

Certain nutrients can help the body rid itself of heavy metals like mercury and aluminum. The mineral **silica** is known to protect the body against aluminum toxicity. Silica is available as a supplement and is extracted from the herb horsetail. I take a mineral in solution formula that contains memory-enhancing B12 plus silica.

In experiments with mice, malic acid—a natural constituent of apples, cherries, and other fruits—effectively removed aluminum from the brains of aluminum-poisoned mice. It worked when taken orally and was even more effective than the chelating drug, deferroxamine, which requires injection and can have toxic side effects. Malic acid may have been the saving force in a fascinating case of Alzheimer's disease involving identical twins.

According to the case report at the 42nd Annual Gerontological Society Meeting in Minneapolis, one of the twins developed Alzheimer's in her early 50s, while her sister was still free of the disease ten years later. This was highly unusual because, in most cases, both identical twins get the disease and, typically, at around the same time.

In this case, the twins lived near each other and were exposed to the same environmental and (with one exception) lifestyle factors. The unaffected twin drank half a bottle of wine a day, while the twin with Alzheimer's did not.

The answer could be the malic acid in wine—a half bottle a day would provide $1\frac{1}{2}$ grams of malic acid, an effective aluminum-chelating dose based on the mouse experiments. Of course, there's no telling what the woman's liver looked like. I wouldn't recommend that we drink half a bottle of wine every day; however, the folk wisdom of eating an apple a day sounds better than ever.

There are other foods that are natural metal-removers. The amino acids cysteine and methionine are especially rich in sulfur. When sulfur combines with hydrogen it makes sulfhydryl groups, which effectively remove toxins and poisons. Foods that are rich in sulfur include onions, garlic, chives, red pepper, and egg yolks. Other excellent sources of sulfur are asparagus, legumes, such as peas, limas, pintos and soybeans, and sesame, pumpkin, sunflower seeds, and English walnuts.

Chelation comes from the Greek word for claw, as in lobster or crab. Medically it is the use of an agent that can claw onto another compound and remove it from the body. A small group of progressive physicians use chelating agents such as EDTA or deferroxamine to bind to calcium or other metals in the bloodstream. This complex is later excreted through urination.

Alzheimer's need not be a worry as you get older; not if you eat well, supplement with all the vitamins and minerals, and replace those ugly silver fillings.

CATARACTS

The eyes are particularly susceptible to pollutants, ultraviolet light, and time. Why? Because they are living tissue not protected by skin. You know how the paint on your car turns white over time? Or how an apple turns brown when cut in half? Or how your curtains fade when exposed to the sun?

These are all processes of oxidation. It's the same process, i.e., free radical damage, that causes cataracts and other degenerative diseases of the eyes. Free radicals are what rust metal and turn bananas brown. Unfortunately, they also gradually break down our bodies over time.

It was the food service industry that first discovered how to retard this process. They needed something that would keep freshly chopped lettuce from becoming unappealingly brown before it could be consumed. They used antioxidants. Some of us use lemon juice (which contains antioxidants) for the same purpose.

Antioxidants are super-duper nutrients that seek out and destroy the free radicals that seek out, ravage, and destroy our skin, joints, tissues, organs, and bones. Fortunately we're constantly discovering new antioxidants all the time. A U.S. Department of Agriculture test identifies foods high in antioxidants and have the ability to quench the free radicals that age us. Called "oxygen radical absorbance capacity" or ORAC, the test determined that the following foods are highest in antioxidant ability: prunes, raisins, blueberries, blackberries, and garlic. I sought out this technology in nutritional supplements and found one formula that uses dehydrated foods to give it the highest ORAC rating of all. A high ORAC rating is the champion, and, therefore, your staunchest ally in your battle against diseases and aging.

Vitamins C and E and beta carotene are the most well-known antioxidants. Others include coenzyme Q-10, selenium, superoxide dismutase (SOD), and the amino acids cysteine, glutathione, methionine, and taurine. Beta carotene is probably the most well-known to date. Everywhere you turn, someone's talking about beta carotene. Believe it or not, scientists have found another biologically occurring nutrient with even more radical-punching ability.

As revealed in a German study on antioxidants, lycopene, a carotenoid flavonoid that is found in the red pigment of the tomato, exhibits the highest oxygen quenching rate of any of the antioxidants. It is also found in tomato products, dried apricots, grapefruit, guava juice, and watermelon.

Want to prevent cataracts? Increase your intake of vitamin E. Among 660 people in a recent Baltimore longitudinal study, those with the most vitamin E in their bloodstreams were 50 percent less likely to develop the most common form of cataracts. The same study that revealed the benefit of lycopene also discovered that alpha tocopherol, or vitamin E, is also a highly effective antioxidant. Take care of your eyes now so your future will have you seeing clearly. Other preventive nutrients include vitamin C with bioflavonoids; vitamin A; the B vitamins thiamine, niacin, riboflavin, and B6; folic acid and biotin.

What's good for the canine is good for the master. Selenium in combination with vitamin E has been used successfully by veterinarians to treat cataracts in dogs. Dogs given these cataract-killers not only lost their cataracts but experienced improved vision as well.

Here's a testimonial for vegetarianism: a 1991 study found that older people who ate a diet of mostly fruits and vegetables were 37 percent less likely to develop cataracts. Many other studies yielded similar results. Look for foods with the crucial cataract-killers. Keep reading and I'll tell you about them. These foods will work miracles against the damaging effects of oxygen on the lenses of the eyes.

A large-scale study of more than 120,000 registered nurses, conducted at Brigham and Women's Hospital and Harvard Medical School, found a 40 percent lower incidence of cataracts among nurses who consumed more foods high in vitamin A as when compared to nurses who consumed less of the same.

Eat your fruits and veggies! If the foregoing didn't convince you, this might. A 1991 report in the *American Journal of Clinical Nutrition* revealed that people who eat 3 1/2 servings of fruits and vegetables every day have a substantially reduced risk of cataracts. Those who ate less than that were believed to be almost six times more at risk for cataracts.

It's a pattern of good eating and supplementation as an effective means of preventing illnesses normally associated with age.

The United States Department of Agriculture agrees. In a study of people who eat less than 1 1/2 servings of fruit or less than two servings of vegetables each day, they determined that those people are roughly 3 1/2 times more likely to develop cataracts.

When researchers questioned the nurses participating in the aforementioned study, they indicated that most of their vitamin A foods were spinach, squash, and sweet potatoes. Yum Yum, some of my favorites!

All orange and dark green vegetables and fruits, as well as fish and cod liver oil, are good food sources of vitamin A. However, vitamin A can be destroyed by poor liver function, alcohol, consuming large quantities of mineral oil or ferrous sulphate (a common preservative found in processed foods), x-rays, and any infection.

Vitamin E is another cataract-killer. This conclusion is also backed by testimony and research from top medical authorities. Studies on vitamin E and cataracts have continually shown that it helps inhibits their development. One eye-opening study (pardon the pun) involving 832 people showed that those with the highest blood levels of vitamin E had the fewest cataracts.

Vitamin C (I never take it without the flavonoids) is probably the most important antioxidant. It not only retards oxidation, but it also reduces inflammation and strengthens the tissues with collagen. There's proof in the pudding! If you mix vitamin C powder with any pureed fruit, it doesn't turn brown.

Experiments with guinea pigs have demonstrated that vitamin C boosts the amount of ascorbic acid in the eyes, helping to stop cataract formation. Researchers have found that the most detectable ascorbic acid (vitamin C) found in the body is in the eyes. The amount of C in the eye is 20 to 70 times higher than levels in the blood and other tissues. By contrast, in eyes with cataracts, very little ascorbic acid is found. In one mind-blowing study, 450 patients who were diagnosed with cataracts experienced a reduction in cataract formation within weeks of taking one gram (1,000 mg) of vitamin C per day.

Ask for whole wheat when you order a sandwich. Why? Because the riboflavin in the wheat can also help fight cataracts, and numerous studies have implicated a deficiency of riboflavin (vitamin B2) in cataract creation. In one study of 173 cataract patients, 20 percent of those under the age of 50, and 34 percent over 50, were deficient in riboflavin. Of the 16 controls over the age of 50 who did not have cataracts, none were deficient in riboflavin. In a study reported in the *Lancet*, eight of 22 cataract patients were determined to be riboflavin deficient. In another study, 81 percent of cataract patients, aged 48-80, had a riboflavin deficiency.

The riboflavin evidence is just the tip of the proverbial iceberg. The amino acid glutathione is found in high concentrations in the cornea and lens of the eye, and keeps the lens transparent, thereby protecting against cataracts. Glutathione protects the lens from the destructive effects of ultraviolet light and is dependent on riboflavin for its production. Glutathione concentration also decreases when the body produces less of the amino acids necessary for its synthesis: cysteine and methionine. And, as I've already mentioned, they, too, are antioxidants!

Glutathione is found in fresh green, yellow, and red vegetables. On the other hand, canned or frozen vegetables lose glutathione during processing. Stay with the fresh stuff. You'll get a lot more out of it.

Another recommended antioxidant, selenium, was found to be only 15 percent of normal levels in the lenses of patients with cataracts. Not coincidentally, selenium also is required for the functioning of glutathione.

Again, we have optimal nutrition, with an emphasis on specific antioxidant nutrients, as the key to prevention. At this point, you should have discerned a pattern. It's a pattern of good eating and supplementation as an effective means of preventing illnesses normally associated with age.

CANCER PREVENTION

As a rule of thumb, eating primarily fruits and vegetables, in addition to high fiber whole grains, will go a long way toward protecting you from cancer. This is a subject I have been researching since the 1960s. I have written two books on the subject, *Nutrition: The Cancer Answer*, and *Nutrition: The Cancer Answer II*. If I may give myself a "pat on the back," I must tell you that I was espousing the virtues of nutrition as a cancer inhibitor long before it was considered a "mainstream philosophy." In the 12 chapters of my book *All Your Health Questions Answered Naturally*, I list specific nutritional regimens for each cancer.

For example, vitamin C and bioflavonoids in berries, cantaloupes, citrus fruits, and green leafy vegetables protect us against cancers of the cervix, the esophagus, and stomach, and vitamin E in wheat germ, nuts, and whole grains guards us against cancers of the breast, pancreas, and stomach.

Antioxidant vitamins C and E, and beta carotene in vegetables and fruits protect cells from damage by free radicals, cell saboteurs that have long been suspected of triggering various cancers. Selenium, a mineral antioxidant, combined with the other minerals, is a power-house in cancer prevention and reversal.

Researchers believe folic acid, one of the B vitamins, may help turn off cancer genes. One study found that a high intake of folic acid, from fresh vegetables and fruit and vitamin supplements, lowered the risk of tumor development. Other research shows folic acid directs the growth of new cells in the body, and a deficiency may contribute to improper or abnormal cell formation.

One of the newer "superstar" anti-cancer nutrients now in supplement form is quercetin, a bioflavonoid. Quercetin is one of the strongest known anti-cancer agents. Various lab studies reveal that quercetin unleashes a one-two punch against cancer. It blocks cell changes that invite cancer and, if a tumor has already started, it stops the spread of malignant cells. Red and yellow onions contain incredible levels of quercetin—10 percent or more of their dry weight.

Adding to what we know about cancer and nutrients, scientists have isolated and identified the many healing chemicals contained in fruits and vegetables. They are collectively called phytochemicals ("phyto" is derived from the Greek word for plant).

Phytochemicals are neither vitamins nor minerals, yet they are equally potent and vital to the healthy functioning of our bodies. They are isolated from plants and are known technically as anthocyanosides, limonoids, glucarates, phenolic acids, flavonoids, coumarins, polyacetylenes, and carotenoids.

Many of mainstream medicine's pharmaceuticals are derived or synthesized from phytochemicals, including aspirin from willow bark and an anti-cancer medication from the Pacific Yew tree.

Broccoli, cauliflower, Brussels sprouts, turnips, chard, kale, turnip greens, and bok choy are the most highly regarded anti-cancer foods. Researchers have isolated a chemical in them called sulforaphane as being most responsible for their cancer preventive properties.

Other foods containing anti-carcinogenic phytochemicals are tomatoes, onions, garlic, turnips, cabbage, strawberries, grapes, raspberries, soybeans, pineapple, sweet potatoes, millet, and almonds. The seeds of every food except citrus contain cancer-blocking agents. Raw apricot kernels, or seeds, contain the most effective phytochemical, amygdalin. In certain studies, amygdalin has been used to not only prevent, but in some cases actually reverse the spread of cancer.

A SEISMIC SHIFT IN HEART CARE

I've been telling people for years that the medical establishment is wrong when it credits cholesterol as the main factor for heart attacks. Some people with high cholesterol live perfectly healthy lives, with no heart disease (If the medical establishment can leave them alone and not push dangerous cholesterol-lowering drugs). And some very sick people, with AIDs, cancer, and heart disease, can have very low cholesterol The secret is now out of the closet and has finally come to light: high cholesterol does not mean sickness, and low cholesterol does not mean health. (Cholesterol is so important to the body that if your cholesterol is too low you have an increased risk of mood disorders, depression, stroke, and violence. Studies have shown a rise in violent deaths among people taking cholesterol-lowering drugs.)

"Revolutionary finding puts inflammation—not cholesterol—as the top risk factor for heart attacks," read one newspaper headline. "It means we have an entire other way of treating, targeting, and preventing heart disease that was essentially missed because of our focus solely on cholesterol," stated Dr. Paul Ridker of Boston's Brigham and Women's Hospital.

I learned this premise years ago as I read the brilliant work of Dr. Valentin Fuster, President of the American Heart Association and director of the Cardiovascular Institute at Mount Sinai School of Medicine in New York. In his book, *The Vulnerable Atherosclerotic Plaque*, he states that high cholesterol is not the only issue of importance.

Many credit heart disease to our poor diets. Make sure your heart muscle is healthy and doesn't have a lot of fat around it.

Inflammation in the circulating blood may play an important role in triggering heart attacks and strokes by activating blood-clotting mechanisms, which in turn can slow down or stop blood flow. Inflammation is the body's natural response to injury, and blood clotting is often part of that response.

A decades-long cycle of irritation, injury, healing, and reinjury to the inside of the blood vessels can cause small arterial plaque deposits to suddenly rupture like popcorn kernels, choking off the blood supply to the heart. The plaque itself can become inflamed as white blood cells invade in a misguided defense attempt. Obesity can contribute to inflammation as fat cells churn out inflammatory proteins.

During the inflammatory process, substance-C-reactive protein is produced in the blood. By measuring blood levels of C-reactive protein, researchers now have an important tool for studying the role of inflammation in heart attacks and strokes, since the amount of inflammation can be measured by the C-reactive protein.

Ridker's 2002 study at Brigham and Women's Hospital showed that measuring C-reactive protein levels can help predict the risk of heart attack in postmenopausal women. In 2001, Brigham researchers showed that C-reactive protein was an excellent way to gauge the heart attack risk in a group of middle-aged men.

Inflammation can be measured with a generic $10 test that looks for high levels of a chemical called C-reactive protein, one of many that increase during inflammation. Dr. Ridker estimates that between 25 million and 35 million healthy middle-aged Americans have normal cholesterol but above-average inflammation.

WHAT YOU CAN DO TO PREVENT HEART ATTACKS

There are two issues to address regarding the prevention of heart problems. One is making sure that your heart muscle is healthy and doesn't have a lot of fat around it. Exercise and certain nutrients will do that. The other is good blood circulation. Exercise also assists in this area.

As described in the previous chapter, inflammation can be overcome by enzymes. For healthy blood and arteries, choose a formula of enterically coated enzymes so they enter the bloodstream instead of being absorbed in the stomach, mimicking the benefits of the enyzme-packed fresh fruits and vegetables recommended by all heart experts.

Many credit our country's high rate of heart disease to our poor diets. Margarine and other hydrogenated trans fats are decidedly not heart smart. Neither is our tradition of eating big meals that include fatty meat. Lean is in—from the tummy to the table.

Generally, any food that improves circulation, has enzymes and nutrients, lowers blood pressure, or causes you to lose weight is going to help prevent heart disease and its complications.

Amino acids, especially L-arginine, will enhance circulation.

In one study, 41 patients with peripheral artery disease consumed a food supplement containing L-arginine and soy protein every day for two weeks. The lucky subjects experienced pain-free walking for a 66 percent longer distance than before treatment, and a 20 percent improvement in total walking distance.

For full supplemental benefit, look for a formula that includes all the amino acids. Amino acids are like the slats of a barrel. You need the full set, and one is only as effective as the shortest slat. Your amino acid formula should be derived from natural sources and include tryptophan. If it is naturally derived, the FDA can't force it off the shelves.

Potassium helps regulate blood pressure and may prevent strokes. A deficiency of this mineral is associated with irregular heartbeat and heart muscle damage. Foods high in potassium are blackstrap molasses, whole grains, dried fruits, avocado, and sunflower seeds.

A deficiency of the mineral copper has been associated with aneurysms (ruptures of the artery) because copper is important for blood vessel strength and elasticity. Foods high in copper are seafood, nuts, beans, peas, molasses, and raisins. Copper supplementation must include zinc. All the minerals work best when taken together in solution.

Olive oil is the reason cited for the low rate of heart disease of people from the Mediterranean. This is because it is an essential fatty acid, which keeps the bad fats out of the arteries. Almonds also contain this good type of fat.

Like the highly touted aspirin, vitamin E acts as a blood thinner, helping to prevent heart attacks. Unlike aspirin, it doesn't cause ulcers. Regular use of aspirin or other non-steroidal, anti-inflammatory painkillers (NSAIDs), such as ibuprofen and naproxen, cause gastric hemorrhage, resulting in about 20,000 deaths yearly. Studies have shown that antioxidants can help prevent damage to the heart muscles after a heart attack as well.

When my friends call to ask advice about a planned surgery, I tell them to take chondroitin sulfate. Clinical studies have shown that chondroitin sulfate works better than Heparin in preventing blood clots (thrombosis) and without the dangerous side effects.

The most potent antioxidant for the heart, coenzyme Q10, is found in beef heart, codfish, egg yolk, mackerel, muscle meat, salmon, sardines, wheat germ, and whole grains.

Selenium, magnesium, and vitamin E in combination have been used successfully in reducing or eliminating recurrent angina attacks (spasms of the heart's coronary artery).

Researchers were perplexed by a lack of heart disease among Europeans who ate a lot of meat and potatoes, until they realized their diets also included foods rich in antioxidants. These foods appeared to offset the damage. Europeans also eat grain-heavy breads. Whole grains are high in muscle-strengthening magnesium and stress-reducing B vitamins.

Deaths due to heart attacks are now believed to be caused by a deficiency of the mineral magnesium. Magnesium requirements are markedly increased during physical stress, and the heart is much more susceptible to arrhythmias during physical exertion if the body's magnesium level is low. Take it in a complete mineral formula in solution for efficient delivery to the cells. Foods high in heart healthy magnesium are whole wheat, pumpkin seeds, millet, almonds, Brazil nuts and hazel nuts, dark-green vegetables, and molasses.

By now it should be obvious that healthy and long living means healthy eating. You are what you ingest, digest, and expect, as well as what you have inherited. Eat wholesome foods, supplement with complete nutrition, and for special problems target certain nutrients. Make sure the nutrients in your supplements are naturally derived, not chemically synthesized. Read on to discover just how important your expectations are to the health of your body.

6

"Is there a split between mind and body? If so, which is better to have?"

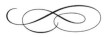

WOODY ALLEN

CHAPTER SIX

THE MIND METER

A Healthy Mind for a Healthy Body

ost of us persist in thinking of mind and body as two separate entities, as though one could exist without the other. The sooner you lose that misconception, the sooner you will gain control over your health and body.

MOST OF US PERSIST IN THINKING of mind and body as two separate entities, as though one could exist without the other. The sooner you lose that misconception, the sooner you will gain control over your health and body.

The fact is, you can "will" yourself to health, youth, and vitality. You can reverse age, disease, and illness just by knowing you can.

The great baseball player Satchel Paige liked to ask, "How old would you be if you didn't know how old you were?" Satch was not a gerontologist, but he was the oldest rookie (age 48) in the history of major league baseball. He understood that age is a state of mind. The same can be true about health and disease.

For the past 25 years researchers have been delving into the mind-body connection trying to answer the question, how does the mind influence the body and vice versa? This is the field of psychoneuroimmunology: psycho (mind) neuro (nervous system) and immunology (study of the immune system), which defines the three-way link between our minds, including thoughts and emotions, our nervous system, and our immune system.

MOLECULES OF EMOTION

Anyone who's ever had a scary thought and felt their heart thump in their chest, or the hair on the back of their neck rise, or literally got cold feet has experienced thought's effect on the body. It isn't surprising that the mind can make you ill. We are more vulnerable to illness when we are under stress. The fact is psychoneuroimmunology, or PNI, represents nothing less than a total revolution in medicine.

Consider the "placebo effect." This is a term used by researchers to describe how some people can be cured of serious diseases by the expectation of being healed—nothing else. When pharmaceutical companies do human studies on their medicines, they have to give some of the patients dummy pills just to statistically eliminate from the statistics the large number of people who can heal themselves.

You didn't have to go to a doctor to grow up. Wounds close themselves, new skin grows, muscles repair, all without medical intervention. In one study, 70 percent of patients improved as a result of "treatments" that were later found ineffective. That's 70 percent of test subjects curing themselves of ailments without medical intervention.

One physician even went so far as to suggest that doctors give their patients dummy pills before prescribing pharmaceuticals with potentially dangerous side effects. The bottom line is (and now even conventional science concurs) that by way of our thought processes alone we have the power to reverse sickness and restore health.

EMOTIONS AND IMMUNE FUNCTION

A large body of research has been amassed that demonstrates a clear link between emotions and the ability of the body to resist disease. Many gerontologists consider aging as nothing more than a collection of diseases and pathologies, and that by resisting disease you are also resisting aging.

Dr. Marvin Stein, a psychiatrist at New York's Mount Sinai School of Medicine, found that bereaved men and severely depressed individuals had fewer disease-fighting white blood cells, called lymphocytes. In a follow-up study, he also found that the immune effects of depression worsened with age. While a group of depressed younger men had normal immune responses, the depressed middle-aged or older patients had declines in two types of lymphocytes—helper T-cells—that fight off viruses and bacteria and natural killer cells that destroy cancer cells.

Not only do brain chemicals circulate freely throughout the body, but the immune system, itself, has a brain. The cells of the immune system are intelligent. They can learn and remember.

Robert Ader, Ph.D., often called the father of neuroimmunology, revealed the learning power of the immune system through a series of experiments in which he was able to stimulate or suppress the immune system of rats by using the power of the conditioned reflex.

This concept was first introduced by the psychologist Pavlov, who was able to induce his dog to salivate at the ring of a bell. In one of Dr. Ader's experiments, he gave rats an immune-suppressing drug flavored with saccharin. By doing this repeatedly, he "taught" the immune system of the rats to suppress its own functioning, even when they were given saccharin without the drug.

Conditioning is a powerful bridge between mind and body, for the body cannot tell the difference between events that are real threats to survival and events that are present in thought alone. In other words, perception becomes reality.

FOOLING THE BODY

Despite a mountain of studies demonstrating that the mind has a powerful influence over the body, much of medical orthodoxy clings to the dinosaur concept that the body and mind are separate, disclaiming or at least discounting the evidence that stress and positive thinking influence the body.

You can will yourself to health, youth, and vitality. You can reverse age, disease, and illness just by knowing you can.

As a species, we are incredibly suggestible. And here is further proof of this. During an athletic event in a stadium in the Southern California city of Highland Park, six people found themselves feeling sick. They crowded into the tiny first aid office complaining of dizziness and nausea.

The nurse questioned them and found they had one thing in common: they all had had a soft drink from the stadium's single vending machine.

Quickly, she phoned an emergency doctor who rushed to the scene and, after talking to the nurse, announced over the public address system no one should use the beverage vending machine or finish any drink taken from it. He told the crowd six people who had drunk a soft drink from it were being treated for dizziness and nausea.

Within five minutes, 200 more people crowded the corridor outside the room. All of them were dizzy and felt like vomiting. The nurse phoned for ambulances.

The ambulances came, were packed with people, and, tires screeching, raced them to the seven nearest hospitals.

Meanwhile, an expert examined the vending machine, its pipes, water source, and soft drink syrup. He found nothing amiss and reported this to the doctor. The doctor announced, via the public address system, that it was all right to use the vending machine. Then he phoned the hospitals to inform stadium patients that a careful examination had revealed that there was nothing wrong with the beverages from the vending machine after all. Within 10 minutes, all the "victims'" symptoms disappeared, and they were released.

How, you may ask, do we overcome a lifetime in which we have been conditioned to believe we need medicine to get well? I rejoice in my healing and praise God for it before it becomes a fact. My belief in God is far stronger than my belief in pharmaceutical medicine and pills. I have witnessed remarkable divine healings. God promises we will be healed and I believe Him. God promises, "No good thing will He withhold from them that walk uprightly."

The God who loves us infinitely cares about our deepest concerns. We have a God who comforts us in grief, provides for our needs, and heals our diseases. "Beloved, I wish above all things that thou mayest prosper and be in health, even as thy soul prospereth" (3 John 1:2).

For those of you who don't have strong faith in God, here are some exercises that will help you make the mind/body connection.

The first one is "imaging." Since the body cannot tell the difference between a real pill and an imagined one, you can fool it by imagining your cure. Let's say you have terrible headaches. Bear in mind, this technique isn't going to work overnight. It takes time for the mind to habitualize the concept so that the body will believe it. Imagine taking a medicine so strong it will kill the worst pain possible. If a particular color works for you, imagine the pill being that color. Now, imagine the pain as a blue cloud moving away from you as healthy sunshine enters your body.

Use whatever pleasure images work for you. Find your pleasure place, a place of faith where you draw comfort, security, and omnipotence, and where you are comfortable and pain-free. Imagine your faith is the pure heavenly light of God driving the pain from your body, or being taken from your body. Or, if you prefer to think literally, picture your brain and the spot on your head that hurts. Imagine that headache as a red, hot glowing spot on your brain. Then imagine your faith dousing it with cool blue water and the redness going away. You get the idea. This has worked for a great many people, and is an excellent example of using the mind and faith to heal the body.

THE POWER OF NOW

*"Take therefore no thought for the morrow:
for the morrow shall take thought for the things of itself.
Sufficient unto the day is the evil thereof."*
MATTHEW 6:34 (NEW TESTAMENT)

A friend recommended a book I thought worthy of mentioning here. It's called *The Power of Now* by Eckhart Tolle (New World Library, Novato, Calif., 1999). He makes the Biblical point that as long as we worry about the past and the future, we are unable to enjoy, appreciate, and fully "seize the moments" of today. We know that negativism creates sickness and we know that optimism encourages health. One way in which to be optimistic is to not dwell on the pains of the past and the worries of the future. Worrying about anything will not change its outcome.

Taking life one day at a time is not only good advice, it's a life saver. If you look at your calendar and contemplate all the appointments, meetings, chores, and deadlines coming up, you'll make yourself crazy—and sick. But if you look at just today and think how quickly it will be resolved, you will retain the vitality, health, and strength necessary to not only cope, but live life more fully.

STRESS AND COPING

It is not stress that counts, but how you feel about it and deal with it. Your attitude, emotional state, and belief can affect your health and ability to deal with every chronic illness, either positively or negatively. Simply put: Upbeat people and people of faith stay healthier, and when they become ill, they handle it better and live longer.

Have you ever had one of those days where you're vacuuming the house, dressing the kids, writing a business proposal, paying the bills, getting the groceries, then getting back into the car and finding that it won't start, and the roof is starting to leak, and on and on? Stress is one mind-body effect that most of us know only too well. Even though stress is a key contributor to almost every illness, from headaches to heart attacks, it need not bring you down. Remember, it is how you cope with stress that determines whether you will be taken ill or feel great. In some studies, people who had a strong belief in God and saw Him working together for good in every circumstance of their lives came through the stress both physically and mentally unscathed. I have a little sign that says, "Your future is as bright as the promises of God." My Bible contains over 7,000 promises. As I claim those promises for my life, accepting that they come from a God who doesn't lie, I gain the peace that surpasses understanding (which God's Word promises).

Just listen to the great world-class athletes who are interviewed during the Olympics. They almost never talk about their problems training for the event, but about the challenges they have had to meet. People who are successful in business or in any kind of endeavor are the same way, thinking of any difficulty they must confront not as a "problem," but a "challenge." You can enjoy challenges, rise to meet challenges, and conquer challenges. Dealing effectively with the stresses in your life increases your sense of competence and enhances health. Prayer, meditation, and relaxation techniques reduce stress, prevent illness, and promote healing. On the other hand, trying to escape stress through substance abuse will only hasten disease and shorten life.

Our thought processes alone have the power to reverse sickness and restore health.

A friend of mine is a very successful entrepreneur who started his own business and now heads a company that grosses in $55 million a year. He told me about his experience with a highly recommended cardiologist.

"Maureen, it was horrible," he lamented. "He spent about five minutes with me, using medical terms so loosely that his words were as incomprehensible to me as Greek. Then he scheduled me for a series of diagnostic tests, each one of which was worse than the other.

"When the tests were over, I went back to the doctor, who read off a series of numbers from the tests in this bored voice. I had such a sense of helplessness, I couldn't even ask him all the questions that I had prepared for my visit. All I kept thinking was, 'Doctor, just tell me what I can do to save my life.'"

There are times when conventional medical treatment can turn the most supremely self-confident individual (like my friend) into a blubbering infant. The feelings of depression, despair, and helplessness that accompany being a passive, infantilized, powerless "patient" can actually worsen illness and hasten death. This is why, on every television show, article, or book chapter, I empower people with hope, awareness, and, most importantly, the knowledge that they can make a difference in their lives.

Patients in the healing process who team with their doctors

are empowered and gain a sense of control that can banish helplessness even in the face of a life-threatening disease. It is widely believed that cancer patients who are actively involved in their healing are more apt to recover than those who become resigned to it. The same is true of heart patients. In the case of my entrepreneur friend in the above story, he thoroughly studied my books, starting with *Nutrition: The Cancer Answer*, then *All Your Health Questions Answered Naturally*, then went on a program of diet, supplementation, exercise, and relaxation exercises that not only restored his health but made him feel decades younger.

FORGIVING THE PAIN FOR A BETTER LIFE

"For if ye forgive men their trespasses, your heavenly Father
will also forgive you. But if ye forgive not men their trespasses,
neither will your Father forgive your trespasses."
MATTHEW 6:14-15

The ability to forgive is more than just a virtue. It is a valuable tool in the search for a better life. It's not a global movement or a meaningless ritual. Forgiveness is personal, a relevation born from a *personal* need to be free from the baggage of anger and hate. "Stand fast therefore in the liberty wherewith Christ hath made us free, and be not entangled again with the yoke of bondage" (Galatians 5:1).

At the Stanford Center for Research in Disease Prevention, Frederic Luskin, Ph.D. conducted a study on how the act of forgiving can help people move past anger, pain, and trauma, and conversely, how the inability to forgive can have a negative impact on individuals and their relationships.

"When we get hurt, we get hurt not just in our minds but also in our bodies," said Luskin. The more readily we experience anger or hurt, the more our bodies secrete "stress chemicals" that, over time, take a toll. But worst of all, Luskin said, the inability to forgive can distract people from the positive aspects of their lives. "If we have too many things that disturb us or that make us feel tense or uncomfortable, what it really does is rob us of our joy."

The study found that by not harboring grudges the participants became less angry. "Their level of hopefulness for the future also significantly increased, and they even felt more spiritual," Luskin said.

The typical study participant showed:

- A 22 percent reduction in stress
- A 20 percent increase in optimism
- A 13 percent reduction in anger, considered a significant risk factor in cardiovascular disease
- A 41 percent reduction in the physical symptoms of stress, including backache, muscle aches, dizziness, and stomach upset.

The results were so impressive that successful workshops and classes in forgiveness are now being conducted, and Luskin has written a book, *Forgive for Good*, Harper Collins, December 2001. For information on his workshops and classes, see www.learningtoforgive.com.

Addressing two dozen participants in one of his forgiveness classes, Luskin puts it bluntly: "Why do we allow someone who is nasty to us to rent so much space in our minds? When someone upsets, hurts, or angers you, what can you do to let go of the offense and not carry a grudge?" In his workshops, Dr. Luskin offers the following seven steps to healing:

1. Make a commitment to yourself to do what you have to do in order to feel better. You're worthy of not continuing to suffer just because of someone's actions. Remind yourself that you deserve not to feel so distressed.

2. Understand your goal. Forgiveness does not necessarily mean reconciliation with the person who upset you, though you

may achieve that. What you are after is to feel better. Forgiveness is the peace and understanding that come from blaming who has hurt you less, taking that person's action less personally, and seeing the cost to you of holding your grudge. Your goal is that peace.

3. Get the right perspective on what's going on. Recognize that your emotional distress is coming from the hurt feelings, thoughts, and physical upset that you are suffering now as a result of what has happened, not what the person who has offended you said or did two minutes—or ten years—ago. What the person did is bad enough. If you dwell on it, your distress increases and, besides the offense itself, you have created an additional problem.

4. Practice a simple stress management technique to counter your body's flight or fight response, which is triggered by being upset. Your heart speeds up, your blood pressure rises, your hands get cold, and you can't think straight. To counter these symptoms and regain calm—at the very moment you start to get upset or recall what happened—bring your attention fully to your stomach as you breathe in and out for two slow and deep breaths. Then picture something in your life that is positive and wonderful. This simple technique cuts the stress response and lets you think more clearly about how to deal with the person who offended you.

5. Give up expecting things from other people that they don't want to give you. If you have been seeking emotional support from someone who does not ever provide it, and this has upset you, for example, ask yourself, How many times will I hit my head against the wall of her coldness hoping that she will be different? Quit demanding that the person who has hurt you will change. Quit waiting for that change. Let your expectations go.

6. Put your energy into looking for another way to get your needs met than through the person who has hurt you. If you have been waiting for a loving relationship with an indifferent

parent, for instance, look for a mentor who can provide the love, guidance, and approval that you crave. Instead of mentally replaying your hurt and distress, seek out new ways to help yourself. If you don't get what you need from one person, don't give up. Just try to get it from another.

7. Remember that a life well lived is your best revenge. Instead of focusing on your wounded feelings, and thereby giving the wounder power over you, learn to look for the beauty and kindness around you. Spend time appreciating the good things in your life and remind yourself of pleasant and loving memories. The moment you shift your thoughts like this, the less you will feel hurt by other people's unkindness. You will start to see that the sun still shines, people still fall in love, and beauty still exists everywhere. These things are still there for you.

THOSE WHO FORGAVE

I have rarely been so touched as the Sunday I took time out of my busy schedule to attend International Forgiveness Day (August 5, 2001) at St. Mary's Cathedral in San Francisco. The people I met and the stories I heard stirred my soul. Keynote speaker Dr. Luskin shared his scientific analysis of the benefits of forgiveness, but it was the people who, despite being victimized by others, were able to forgive their trespassers that made the deepest impact on all who attended. As they received a special "Hero of Forgiveness" honor, we learned their stories.

Saundra Adams forgave NFL football star Rae Carruth as he was sentenced to 18 years in prison for the murder of her daughter, Cherica. Pregnant with Carruth's child when she was gunned down by a hired assassin, Cherica underwent an emergency Caesarean section hours after the shooting. She died almost a month later. Saundra is now raising her grandson, who has cerebral palsy. Said Saundra, "I forgave because God forgave me. I didn't feel like forgiving, but I made the decision to forgive because I wanted to be the type of person I want my grandson to be."

In 1978, at the impressionable age of 11, Timothy Streett witnessed the brutal murder of his beloved father, a retired Army chaplain who had survived the horrors of Vietnam. The murder took place in a tough Detroit neighborhood. Cleaning snow from the driveway, a gang of boys descended on Timothy and his father. His father asked, "What's going on?" They demanded what they had, which was one dollar. One of the boys blasted Timothy's father with a bullet in the heart.

The ability to forgive is more than just a virtue. It is a valuable tool in the search for a better life.

Timothy lived through this horrible experience and as an adult realized what his father would do. He became determined to embrace the healing of forgiveness. Timothy went to establish a sports ministry in the neighborhood in which his father's murderers had grown up. He found his father's murderer, forgave him, and befriended his family and the rest of the gang. Said Tim of the attention he has received as a result of his selfless acts, "I have done so little, but I have a God that has done so much."

"The enemy taught me how to love myself," said Paul Reed, a U.S. Veteran of the Vietnam War. In one battle, Reed saw many of his courageous friends, who had formed a brotherhood during the conflict, riddled to shreds by sniper bullets fired by a contingent of Vietnamese soldiers. One of the Vietnamese—a man named Nguyen van Nghia—Reed thought he had killed. Tormented by the experience for decades, a thoughtful friend reminded Reed that he had Nghia's diary, which Reed had taken from the lifeless body as a souvenir.

For the first time in 20 years, Reed opened the diary and found Nghia's picture. Curious, he had it translated and discovered his enemy's humanity. Inside was beautiful poetry written by Nghia, to his wife, expressing his desire to be home again. Touched, Reed sought out Nghia's family. He discovered Nghia was not dead, but was partially blinded. They met and forgave each other. Then, in an incredible act of not only forgiveness but benevolence, Reed brought Nghia to the U.S. for the partial restoration of the eyesight he lost during that fateful battle. I'll never forget Paul's insightful analogy of forgiveness. A former paratrooper, he likened forgiveness to the release of a parachute after a jump. "You release the straps so you don't get dragged to death."

When I think of those I must forgive, I think of how small my grudges are, as compared to these people who have forgiven so much. When Jesus said, "Love one another," the definition of love (there are nine in the Koina Greek) means no vindictiveness, no bitterness, no jealousy, no anger or rancor. "Thou shalt not avenge, nor bear any grudge against the children of thy people, but thou shalt love thy neighbour as thyself" (Leviticus 19:18).

The Reverend Karyl Huntley helped define forgiveness. She said, "How I know if I have forgiven someone is that he or she has safe passage in my mind."

NUTRITIONAL SOLUTIONS TO STRESS

If an ounce of prevention is worth a pound of cure, as it relates to stress, then vitamin E is worth its weight in plutonium.

Researchers in Sweden and Cairo found that when they gave vitamin E to rats before subjecting them to stress, the vitamin normalized the metabolism of the brain and protected it against the harmful effects of stress hormones. Indeed, taking vitamin E was almost as effective in reducing stress as Valium, the anti-anxiety drug with which it was compared.

Earlier studies had shown that stress from many different sources, such as noise or emotional turmoil, increases the production of free radicals. Vitamin E, a powerful antioxidant, was able to retard free radical formation and prevent stress-induced chemical changes in brain metabolism.

Recently, a young working woman complained that she was anxious, irritable, and having trouble sleeping. It sounded like the classic symptoms of stress. When I asked what her daily diet consisted of, she told me that she starts the day with coffee and a Danish at her desk, often skips lunch because she's "watching her weight," and then wolfs down a microwaved frozen meal while she zones out in front of the TV. And she wonders why she experiences stress!

My friend is giving herself a double whammy. Not only is she failing to supply herself with the nutrients she needs to combat stress, but the stress itself is depleting her body of nutrients, particularly magnesium. Stress causes a stimulation of the adrenal hormones, which in turn causes the body to lose magnesium.

Other factors that contribute to magnesium deficiency are foods like white bread, highly sweetened desserts (from which magnesium has been removed in the processing), and alcohol, which increases the loss of the mineral in the urine.

Magnesium acts like a natural tranquilizer, calming the nervous system and protecting the heart and other muscles. A friend of mine had panic attacks as well as mitral valve prolapse, a heart condition in which some blood leaks through the valve and causes palpitations or fluttering of the heart. My husband, the late Dr. Ross Gordon, put her on 600 mg of magnesium in divided doses, and a month later she informed him that her panic attacks and anxiety had vanished and her palpitations were almost gone.

Stress can be the body's signal that it's not getting the nutrients it needs. Often symptoms of stress, such as anxiety, depression, allergic-like reactions, food and chemical intolerances, and hyperactivity can be explained by a careful examination of diet, as well as vitamin, mineral, enzyme, and other nutrient levels.

Stress causes more vitamins and minerals to be taken from the body. Support your stress mechanism by supplementing with additional vitamins and minerals.

If you suspect your stress is diet-related, eliminate caffeine and food additives from your diet and eat fresh, whole foods, high in carbohydrates, low in fat, and moderate in protein. Less than two per cent of the diet should come from simple sugars.

I've found that a primarily vegetarian diet (that includes occasional servings of fish, but no milk products because I'm allergic) with appropriate supplementation has completely relieved me of periodic stress "wipeouts." The stress reaction also interferes with digestion and the absorption of vitamins and minerals by the cells and into tissues. Nutrients can protect and aid the body in stressful times, building up the immune system, thereby helping you withstand stress, tension, and anxiety.

In highly stressful situations, I recommend the following supplements: B-complex vitamins, particularly pantothenic acid, 500 mg (three times daily) of vitamin C with bioflavonoids, 800 IUs of vitamin E, an amino acid formula that contains tyrosine and tryptophan (these produce a calming effect on the nervous system), and a good mineral (in solution) formula that contains vitamin B12 and more magnesium than calcium, i.e., in a three or four to one ratio.

You can give yourself control of your health. Properly supplementing your diet can help reduce or eliminate stress's negative impact on the body.

POWER TOOLS OF THE BRAIN

You don't have to "fool your mind" to trick your body into good health. You can pick up the brain's power tools and use them at will to control your ability to resist and recover from disease, thereby promoting youthfulness and longevity. The tools I use are faith healing, prayer, positive thinking, and an optimistic attitude, which also emanates from my faith. Other tools of mind over body include hypnosis, autosuggestion, and biofeedback.

Begin by making your health your responsibility rather than abdicating to doctors and hospitals, and remember that you are not alone. Rather, you are joining an ever-growing movement of empowered patient/consumers, seeking out alternative therapies and medicine, and reestablishing control of their own lives and health. Most importantly, don't forget that you are the senior partner in your personal health care firm, and that your doctor is only the junior partner.

The mind has a powerful influence over the body to fight off aging and disease.

Taking responsibility means making greater demands of yourself. This is a blessing in disguise. Studies show increasing the mental demands of elderly people increases their longevity. In a study of arthritis patients who were given stimulating mental activity like word puzzles, it was determined that, when compared with the group given less stimulating tests, the intellectually challenged patients reported feeling increased levels of comfort and enjoyment. In some cases, the positive mental activity even helped their arthritis!

THE BRAIN GAIN

If you have a garden, you know you can actively encourage new growth by pruning and cutting back. The brain grows in much the same way, making new nerve connections to fill in the gaps created by old cells that have died off. This resprouting, or "reactive synaptogenesis," keeps the brainpower going even though, by age 90, we may lose up to 40 percent of our nerve-cell connections. Mental challenges nourish and encourage this regrowth, limiting cell loss and keeping the brain young.

Marian Diamond, Ph.D., an anatomist at the University of California in Berkeley, demonstrated that the brains of old rats grew when they were placed in novel situations, such as having their cages filled with toys. The resprouting occurred in areas of the brain associated with learning, memory, and understanding. In case you think this is only a rat story, you should know that Professor Diamond is also famous for having studied Einstein's brain. Arguably the most intelligent man of the 20th Century, Einstein's gray matter turned out to be thickly studded with dendrites, the branchlike connections between the neurons.

We have a God who comforts us in grief, provides for our needs, and heals our diseases.

Stretch that mind, pump those neurons, drive those dendrites. "Use it or lose it" applies as much, or even more, to the brain as to the body. You've got to exercise the old gray matter to keep it young, flexible, and healthy. Research in both animals and people shows that cerebral calisthenics can actually *reverse* age's wear and tear on the brain. In terms of performance levels, brain-training turned back the clock an average of 14 years in two out of five older volunteers.

A National Institute on Aging report found that one in five intellectually impaired old people can actually improve function with brain workouts. Studying new things can even boost scores on standard mental function tests, enabling older people to perform more like their younger counterparts.

New situations place stress on us, but this can work to our benefit rather than to our detriment. In one experiment, rats were placed into a new (stressful) situation on a daily basis. Every day they had to find new food and make up a new nest. Instead of falling apart from the stress, they stayed young, lean, muscular, and vital to a much prolonged old age. The rats that had everything provided for them became placid, doddering, and lost their youthful curiosity and enthusiasm.

Controlling one's destiny by accepting life's challenges boosts immune function and fights cancer. In another experiment, rats given control over whether they could escape unpleasant stimuli were better able to reject injected tumor cells, while rats conditioned to helplessness developed cancer from the tumors and died earlier.

I always serve my audiences by raising their T cells. When I stand before them, I can see their thinking in their eyes: "Give me the hope to go on." I always do! There is no such thing as false hope. Hope is hope with all its spirit-elevating elements. Positive expectations are the rungs on the ladder that lead to hope. What makes you grow old is replacing hope with regret.

WATCH YOUR LANGUAGE

When Barbara Levine was 32, she was stricken with a massive, life-threatening brain tumor. Like many other dreadfully ill people, she had to endure years of misdiagnoses and hundreds of tests, but then she did something no other patient had. She spent the next 15 years researching how our language, the words we use daily without a moment's reflection, can physically harm or heal our body. The result was a complete recovery and a book, *Your Body Believes Every Word You Say.*

Seemingly innocuous phrases and images like "pain in the neck," "it comes right out of my hide," and "that breaks my heart" are what Levine calls "seedthoughts" that can lead to the larger plants of illness and dysfunction. Listen to what you say, she urges, and choose your words and images wisely. She contends the words you utter can actually change the course of disease.

Be aware of clichés and other expressions that may unconsciously sow negative thoughts. Practicing this "verbal hygiene," as she calls it, will keep you from passing on negative messages to yourself and others.

In one dramatic example of this phenomenon, Alice, a friend

of mine who has long suffered from asthma, told me what it was like growing up in her family. "My parents were so overbearing," she said. "They always wanted to know where I went, what I did, what I was thinking at that very moment. Their love was suffocating to me. I couldn't breathe." Until I pointed it out to her, Alice had never made the connection between those words (which she had often used to herself) and her asthma symptoms.

What we tell ourselves also has a direct bearing on how rapidly we age. The next time you think or say out loud, "I'm too old for. . ." skiing, horseback riding, learning to play piano, or whatever, change it to "I'm still young enough for that." As another friend of mine likes to say whenever someone complains "life's too short for. . ." arguing, working long hours, putting up with one's boss, etc., that instead one should say, "Life is too long not to make every moment work for you."

The Bible also has a great deal to say about the power of our words. *"Death and life are in the power of the tongue"* (Proverbs 18:21).

Words are serious business. We need to get serious about learning how to use them. We need to begin to put them to work for us. As Apostle Paul said in 2 Corinthians 4:13, *"We have the same spirit of faith as he had who wrote, 'I believed, and therefore have I spoken. We too believe, and therefore we speak' "* (AMP).

Words won't work without faith any more than faith will work without words. It takes both to put the law of results in motion. If you speak the words but don't yet believe them, take heart. If you speak the words often enough, the subconscious mind will come to believe them. You'll cross the line from hope to faith, and you'll start seeing those mountains move. It is then that miracles can occur.

PROGRAMMING FOR THE NEXT 100 YEARS

There is a conspiracy that surrounds you. It is in the newspapers, magazines, and books you read, the TV and films you watch, the people you talk to, the doctors you may visit, even the greeting cards that you send and receive. Everything in the culture passes on the message: after age 50 or thereabouts, you are getting older, sicker, weaker, and closer to death with each passing year.

On TV shows where a person in his 70s is shown playing golf or performing some other activity, the implication is often "isn't that remarkable for his age?" Our surprise is proof of our low expectations. Mind-body researchers have shown that our expectations, what we *believe* about aging, creates the program for our mind, which in turn influences the body to fulfill these expectations. We expect to go downhill and feel worse with age, therefore we are not surprised when we do.

Upbeat people and people of faith stay healthier, and when they become ill, they handle it better and live longer.

Once you are aware of these negative perceptions and expectations you can get rid of them and reprogram your mind for longevity. Start today by thinking about aging as growth, and expect that each passing year will hold new wonders and delights.

Here are some tips for reprogramming your mental software.

1. Relax in your favorite chair, two or three times each day for about 10 minutes at a time, feet flat on the floor, and imagine yourself at 90, as full of life as you are now.

2. In your mind, create a movie about how you want to feel. Visualize yourself enjoying life, being strong and healthy, surrounded by friends and family who love you and value your wisdom and lifetime of experience.

3. Repeat 20 times in succession, twice daily, a message of affirmation like "Thank you Lord for restoring my soul and body"—an adaptation from Psalms. Caleb did it in the Old Testament. He said, "I am as strong at 90 as I was in my youth."

Time travel is another technique for mental programming. Where do you want to live when you're 90? What would you like to accomplish at age 100? Where would you and your husband or wife or loved one like to travel to in the year 2040? Think about the future, imagine the future, plan to be there, and you will.

BACK TO THE FUTURE

In 1979, Harvard researcher Ellen Langer and her colleagues invited a group of men, age 75 and older, to spend a week at a country resort. They were given one stipulation: leave home anything like a newspaper, magazine, book, or family photo dated later than 1959.

Every detail of their week in the country was set up to duplicate life exactly as it was 20 years earlier. The magazine racks held copies of *Life* and *Saturday Evening Post* dated 1959. The music that was played on the phonograph was two decades old, and the men were instructed to behave as though the year was 1959, speaking only of people and events of that time.

They wore ID photos that had been taken in 1959 and soon learned to identify one another through their pictures rather than their present appearance. They spoke of their wives and children and of the details of their own lives as though they were 20 years younger and still living in 1959. Although all the men were retired, they acted as though their careers were ongoing.

The week's holiday from their present lives made a lasting impression on the men. Compared with a control group that went on the same retreat but continued to live in the year 1979, the time travelers had improved memory and manual dexterity, higher level of activity, and increased self-sufficiency. Although many of them had become dependent on a younger family member to do simple everyday tasks, by the end of the week at the resort, they were taking their own food at meals, cleaning up their rooms, and behaving like middle-aged men.

Perhaps the most remarkable changes had to do with so-called irreversible aspects of aging. Impartial judges asked to study before-and-after photos of the men testified that their faces looked visibly younger by an average of three years. Even their fingers, which typically shrink with age, had lengthened. They had started to straighten up and take the lead out of their joints. Furthermore, they had gotten smarter. Intelligence is considered fixed in adults, yet half the group showed increased intelligence over the five days during which they returned to 1959.

Proving that this was no fluke were the results of a control group who went on the same retreat but continued to live in the year 1979. Although they also experienced some improvement just by going on a trip for a week and being made the object of special attention, their finger length and manual dexterity actually declined, and one-quarter of the control group had lower IQ test scores than when they were tested prior to the retreat.

You don't have to take out your old photos and surround yourself with images and music from 1980 to feel 20 years younger. You can accomplish the same thing as the time voyagers by giving mindful attention to the world around you, becoming aware of hidden negative messages, words, and images that subtly tell you it's all right to be old, to feel creaky and achy, to let the kids take out the garbage or rake the leaves when you're perfectly capable of doing it yourself.

You are not only as young as you feel, you are as young as you do and think. Now is the time for you to raise your personal expectations.

CHAPTER SEVEN

HORMONAL HELPERS

The Newest Anti-Aging Medicine: Natural, Supplemental Hormones

onsidering the enormous popularity and progress of nutritional therapy, it's not hard to predict that enlightenment and a serious rethinking of traditional medicine will occur in the 21st Century. It wasn't that long ago that conventional medicine labeled acupuncture "quack" medicine. Today, many HMO physicians recommend acupuncture for pain relief. Tomorrow it will be supplemental hormones to combat aging.

SCIENTISTS HAVE FINALLY DISCOVERED WHY OUR BODY AGES—why skin wrinkles, muscles convert to fat, bones get thinner, our reactions and thought processes slow, and our eyesight fails. It's many things, including a natural decline in human growth hormone.

Hormonal changes occur naturally, as we age, in both women and men. These changes can cause fatigue, weight gain, insomnia, loss of libido (sex drive), hair loss, loss of skin firmness, brain fog, anxiety, and depression. Many of these symptoms can be relieved or alleviated by balancing the body's system with *natural hormones*.

In women, these problems, along with more classic symptoms such as hot flashes and vaginal dryness, can begin years before the menstrual cycle ends. In both women and men these changes can result from an imbalance of hormones, including estrogen, progesterone, testosterone, DHEA, and thyroid hormone. It is the *change* in the balance of these hormones, not just the fall of any one, that needs to be identified.

A natural hormone is identical in structure and function to hormones produced by the body. The way to add these hormones naturally is to use a soy or yam-based progesterone cream that is absorbed through the skin. A natural hormone program replaces these lost hormones together, not one by one, in order to create balance in the body as a result of age, stress, and nutrient deficiency. This avoids the more common medical practice of using a large dose of only one hormone.

WHAT IS HUMAN GROWTH HORMONE?

If you've heard about human growth hormone (HGH), you might have gotten the impression it's a magic pill to reverse aging. You may believe it's too good to be true and must be quack medicine.

The use of HGH for human afflictions came about through scientific study. It is valid and available. Dr. Denise Mark of Morgan Hill, CA (408-778-3601) is one of the world's experts on hormones. Her clientele come from all over the world to obtain her uniquely expert care. She and the equally expert Dr. Murray Susser and Dr. Richard E. Casdorph have reviewed more research than any of the many doctors I know. Dr. Mark says the research is valid, but what you should know is your body right now is producing HGH. As you grow older, it will produce less. However, there are certain things you can do to increase and/or maintain your body's production of HGH.

Prior to considering a plan of action, don't forget the ABCs of good health and age reversal: good food, a positive attitude, faith in God, and supplementing with minerals, vitamins, amino acids, enzymes, essential fatty acids, and antioxidants.

Technically, human growth hormone is a polypeptide protein with 191 amino acids and a molecular mass of 22 kilodaltons. Since it is an extremely large and complex protein, it is destroyed by stomach acid and the process of digestion.

A natural hormone replaces lost hormones together in order to create balance in the body as a result of age, stress, and nutrient deficiency.

HGH is secreted by specialized cells in the pituitary gland called sematotropes. They are the dominant cell type in the pituitary, making up 50 percent of the pituitary's cells. HGH is released from the pituitary in response to somatotropin (GHRH). HGH is the primary hormone responsible for maintaining physical and mental health through tissue repair, healing, cell replacement, bone strength, brain function, enzyme production, and integrity of hair, nails, and skin.

The pituitary gland is a major organ in the immune system. What triggers the release of the hormone is important to note. I will explain the significance of this later. HGH decreases with age (at a rate of roughly 14 percent per decade of adult life). By the age of 60 it is not uncommon to see declines of 75 percent. Studies have repeatedly shown that about half of all older adults (those over 65) are growth-hormone deficient. Enough hormone is probably being made by the pituitary, but for various reasons the body is not able to utilize it.

THE USE OF HGH IN HUMANS

Human use of HGH began in 1958 when endocrinologist Maurice Rabin injected it into a child with dwarfism. The child began to grow normally, and over the next 30 years thousands of growth-restricted children were treated with HGH. However, many more went without the therapy. At the time, the only way to obtain human growth hormone was to painstakingly extract it from the pituitary glands of human cadavers. There was never enough of the extracted hormone to offer treatment to all the growth hormone-deficient children in the U.S. Furthermore, there was not even enough for conducting necessary research.

Legislation opened up research to develop a synthetic version so all HGH-deficient children could benefit. The pharmaceutical industry responded. In 1985, Genentech developed Protropin. The following year, the drug company Eli Lilly produced a synthetic form identical to natural human growth hormone. Lilly's Humatrope was approved by the FDA for research and medical use—but only for children.

BREAKTHROUGH STUDY
ON HGH FOR AGING

On July 5, 1990, America's most prestigious medical journal, *The New England Journal of Medicine*, published a human clinical study that changed the world of anti-aging medicine forever.

Daniel Rudman, M.D., and colleagues reported the results of their six-month trial study of synthetic human growth hormone with 12 elderly men, aged 61 to 81. Astoundingly, without any change in diet, exercise, lifestyle, smoking etc., the men gained muscle, lost fat, increased their bone density, thickened their skin, and expanded their livers and spleens by almost 20 percent. In effect, HGH reversed the biological age of the subjects by 10 to 20 years.

Taking up the torch, Edmund Chein, M.D., began treating the elderly with HGH. From 1994 to 1996, over 800 people were treated with HGH at Dr. Chein's Palm Springs clinic, the

Life Extension Institute. Chein collaborated with Dr. L. Cass Terry so the mass of clinical data could be turned into meaningful statistical results. Their findings convinced many that HGH can improve the quality of life for many elderly people. They even convinced the FDA. In 1996, the FDA sanctioned the therapeutic use of HGH for adults.

Today, many physicians are treating their patients with HGH therapy. Richard Casdorph, M.D., Ph.D., F.A.C.P, is a highly respected doctor and credentialed physician practicing out of Long Beach, California (562-597-8716). He is brilliant, has excellent credentials, and as a consummate professional, wears many hats: professor, practitioner, and innovative diplomat of the American Board of Internal Medicine. Dr. Casdorph notes that many patients have opted for HGH instead of invasive and risky cosmetic surgery, often achieving the same desirable results. He uses injections, then follows up with oral sprays. He has successfully treated Alzheimer's, Crohn's disease, and other maladies.

Here are some of the benefits experienced by his patients:

- Significant fat loss—fat converts to muscle
- Improvement in skin texture, thickness, elasticity, and disappearance of wrinkles
- New hair growth
- Improved healing of injuries
- Resistance to colds and common illnesses
- Improved sexual functioning
- Increased energy level, stamina
- Less depression, better mood, positive attitude, and increased memory capacity

In addition, subjects have improved cardiovascular health, stronger bones, improved cholesterol levels, lung, kidney, liver and spleen function, and sleep. Casdorph noted that 85 percent of his patients have increased energy within 1-3 months of starting HGH therapy, with additional increases over six months. At that point they seem to plateau. HGH has been shown to be particularly helpful with chronic fatigue syndrome. Noted side effects are uncommon, minor, and temporary. They include water retention and joint pain.

Many of the symptoms of aging can be relieved or alleviated by balancing the body's system with natural hormones.

Dr. Murray Susser, practicing out of West Los Angeles (310-453-4424), has treated several thousand people with various forms of hormone replacement over the course of many years, and he believes that HGH is one of the cornerstones of longevity therapy.

"Growth hormone may be the most sizzling and exciting poster child," says Dr. Susser, "because of its dramatic effect on improving how the proteins in our muscles, bones, and vital organs function and rejuvenate."

Dr. Susser recounts the case history of a patient who was a devoted body builder but had watched his personal best at lifting steadily decline for 20 years. Dr. Susser started him on HGH, and in just over a month he increased his lifting strength by 30 percent—to the level at which he had performed about ten years prior.

The doctor added, "This case history is just about as meaningful to me as a controlled scientific study."

In his practice he uses approximately one unit/day, with a range of about 4-8 units per week, depending on individual needs and tolerance of the hormone. Three units equal one cc. A standard dose is four units a week.

Susser also sees value in amino acid stimulants because they work as secretogogues, stimulating the pituitary gland to secrete more HGH. Researchers have published many studies that demonstrate that the amino acids arginine, ornithine, glutamine, lysine, and methionine can increase the production of HGH.

Dr. Susser measures the patient's IGF-1 (insulin growth factor 1) to determine how well his treatment is working and has found amino acids increase IGF-1 by 50 percent in approximately half the people who had low IGF levels to begin with.

Susser believes that HGH is extremely safe when used in physiologic doses. He questions the concerns some have raised about HGH increasing the growth of various cancers, and makes the following observations as reasons to doubt this theory.

"No study with HGH use has shown any increased risk of cancer," Susser testifies. "HGH use in one form or another has been around for perhaps a half century without any evidence of increased cancer. One can look at the history of its use by body builders, many of whom have clearly overdosed the black market hormone for years, to provide strong evidence that a relatively robust and opposite population from the AIDS patient does not show evidence of increased cancer. AIDS patients are being treated with 18 units per day of HGH. They have the greatest risk of cancer of any population of which I know. Yet, their treatment is about 18 times the amount usually given as a replacement dose and there is no evidence of increased cancer risk in the AIDS patient."

In summary, HGH given in physiologic doses seems to be a safe and effective approach to slowing and even reversing some of the aging process.

WHO NEEDS HGH?

The first adults I would recommend for anti-aging HGH therapy are those whose quality of life has been affected: the elderly and infirm. If it can help someone walk straighter and stronger, feel better about life, and see and think more clearly, I'm all for it. When I think of all the people out there who have been crippled by time, restricted to a wheelchair or their living rooms because of their frailty, I want to scream, "Why?" Primarily because the cost of HGH is prohibitively expensive. So many who could use it can't afford it. One pharmaceutical website lists the cost of six vials of Lilly's Humatrope at $1,500. Many doctors are still ignorant of the facts and discourage patients' use of HGH as a pipe dream. It is unfortunate that the most complete forms have to be purchased at a pharmacy with a doctor's prescription.

Researcher Susan R. Levin of L.I.F.E. Research Clinics is working with the FDA on studies that will, once and for all, make a determination of HGH's effectiveness and in what form. She is working on an injectable, active form, training doctors on how to use it and what it does. She says her scientists state that because "it is ineffective within a short time of being mixed with fluid it is not effective in spray form." Until such time as the studies are complete and manufacturers can catch up, or you are fortunate enough to have doctors like Dr. Mark, Dr. Susser or Dr. Casdorph, the best way to get HGH is to encourage the body to produce it on its own. In the next section I will show you how to do so.

DO YOU NEED HGH?

Physicians who offer HGH therapy conduct tests to determine if their patients are low in human growth hormone. The only way to identify the amount of HGH in the body is to measure the amount of insulin-like growth factor 1 (IGF-1) produced by the liver. Low IGF-1 equals low human growth hormone. In lab lingo, the test for IGF-1 is called a Somatomedin-C test.

If you are having this lab test done, be sure to remind the person taking the blood sample to freeze it immediately. If it is not frozen your result will be worthless. The normal range of IGF-1 is 90-360 ug/ml (as determined by Corning Laboratories in San Diego, CA).

Other tests look at the symptoms of low HGH, including thin skin and poor elasticity, slow reaction times, reduced sweating, sensitivity to cold, obesity, hypertension, lack of sex drive, and chronic dehydration.

Terry Grossman, M.D., conducts a few inexpensive, logical tests to determine biological age, and if patients can be helped with HGH:

• **Reaction Time:** Drop a ruler between patients' fingers and see how many inches it drops before they catch it. Measures reaction time.

• **Near Vision:** See how close the patient has to hold a newspaper to read.

• **Skin elasticity, dehydration:** Pinch the skin on the back of the hand. See how long it takes to go down.

• **Neurological System:** Time how long the patient can stand on one stocking foot, with eyes closed.

• **Fat to Muscle Ratio**

Dr. Grossman uses these simple tests to determine the state of the patient's health, then later the effectiveness of HGH therapy.

HOW TO GET HGH

The best and most reliable way to get HGH is to increase your output naturally. The first way to do this is by not eating before bed. Why? Because the process of digestion interferes with deep sleep, and HGH increases during the deepest part of slumber, REM sleep, when you dream. Do not eat at least two hours before going to bed. Bedtime snacks suppress the release and fat-burning effects of HGH.

Intense physical exercise also increases the production of HGH. So not only does a good workout help you build muscle, but it helps reverse aging.

Since digestion decreases HGH, going without eating, as in fasting, increases it. The best way to increase your natural levels of HGH is to avoid bedtime eating, get plenty of quality sleep, avoid drugs and alcohol, and get regular vigorous exercise that encourages your body to produce HGH. Calcium is a critical mineral in the metabolism of HGH, and a zinc deficiency will reduce the release of HGH. It is recommended that before attempting to increase HGH, you get a hair analysis for heavy metals. The presence of mercury in the body is associated with not only mental illness, but many of the symptoms of aging. Mercury will displace zinc (diminishing wound healing) and bind to HGH, keeping it from being released from the pituitary. Mercury also stops the absorption of magnesium, important to strong muscles and good circulation.

If you are expecting to realize maximum results from HGH, make sure you have good blood levels of minerals, low acid urine (indicative of mineral loss), and have good blood sugar balance. Hormones are complex. If you do not respond, seek out a natural healing doctor and have a blood panel done. A physician can give you guidance on what to do (or not do)—and that can make all the difference.

MELATONIN, DHEA, AND PREGNENOLONE

Hormones are not to be taken lightly by women *or men* when it comes to the aging process. As people age, their hormone levels drop. The key to slowing the aging process is to fool your body into believing you are still young, with the same levels of youthful hormones you always had.

Three hormones directly connected to the immune system drop dramatically with age. They are melatonin, DHEA, and pregnenolone.

Melatonin is a hormone produced by the pineal gland and is

increased in the blood during hours of darkness. In the daytime it is typically found in low concentrations. Melatonin promotes sleep and contributes to the circadian rhythm—the sleep-wake rhythm—and body temperature. It is increased in the blood during hours of darkness.

Have you ever noticed how when you are very tired, you feel cold? Or how warm air can lull you to sleep? This is melatonin at work. Remember, sleep is very important to preventing further aging. It's only during the deepest phases of sleep that human growth hormone is produced. It is called the anti-stress hormone, due to the fact that it regulates the rhythms of other hormones.

Melatonin produces effects that are nearly the mirror image of those caused by bright light. It can work in cases where a lack of light causes seasonal affective disorder or SAD. A decrease in melatonin concentration has been reported in most studies of depressed patients.

The key to slowing the aging process is to fool your body into believing you are still young, with the same levels of youthful hormones you always had.

Other benefits include strengthening the function of the pineal gland, antioxidant and free radical scavenging, influencing thyroid hormone production for adequate energy, calming the digestive tract in order to give our bodies enough time to utilize nutrients, normalizing blood zinc levels, helping to bolster and preserve the efficiency of each primary organ in the body, boosting immunity and strengthening our resistance against infection and cancer, helping to keep cholesterol levels normal and our hearts strong, restoring thymus gland function, and encouraging the body's natural antibody response.

Melatonin's effect on estrogen could also reduce the risk of breast cancer experienced by postmenopausal women. Studies show that melatonin boosts the ability of Tamoxifen to inhibit the growth of human cancer cells in the laboratory.

Walter Pierpaoli, M.D., Ph.D., head of Laboratory and Research at the Biancalana-Masera Foundation for the Aged in Nancona, Italy, conducted an experiment in which elderly mice were given melatonin in their drinking water. Pierpaoli found that melatonin-treated mice lived six months longer (25 human years) than typical mice life expectancy and died not from cancer, like many others, but from aged organs. Other symptoms exhibited by the melatonin-mice were the development of thick, shiny coats, their eyes were cleared of cataracts, and their vigor and strength improved. The experiment was repeated several times with the same results.

In another experiment, young pineal glands were transplanted into old mice. A control group of mice had their old pineals taken out and put back in. The mice with the new pineals "lived an average 30 percent longer and maintained their youthful, vigorous bodies until the very end of life, which was about 33 months, or in human terms, around 105 years."

In his book, *Melatonin Miracle*, Pierpaoli testified that, "Melatonin supplementation helped bring the pineal back to its youthful state, and in doing so altered the message it was sending to the rest of the body and restored normal cyclicity or balance to the body. By taking a very small dose of melatonin, just enough to boost your melatonin level back to what it was when you were in your twenties, you can keep your body and each of its essential systems functioning in the synchronized manner they did in your youth."

Pierpaoli recommends the following dosages:

.5 to 1 mg	ages 40-44
1 to 2 mg	ages 45-54
2 to 2.25 mg	ages 55-64
2.5 to 5 mg	ages 65-74
3.5 to 5 mg	over age 75

Take the lower dosage first, then gradually increase until you get the results you desire.

Melatonin and DHEA (dehydroepiandrosterone) have connections to the adrenals that may prove to be advantageous to menopausal women.

A study reported in the *American Journal of Obstetrical Gynecology* (December 1993) concluded that DHEA may be beneficial to postmenopausal women who exhibit a deficiency of androgens, male hormones produced by the adrenals. Before taking DHEA for a prolonged period of time, I recommend that you see a health care practitioner who is familiar with the use of this hormone. Because DHEA can be converted to potent androgens, such as testosterone, it can cause masculine symptoms in women, including growing facial hair.

Hormones are not to be taken lightly by women or men when it comes to the aging process. As people age, their hormone levels drop.

The researchers also noted the strong T-cell activity of DHEA, suggesting any problem that involves a dysfunction of the adrenals could be remedied by DHEA, including uterine and breast cancer, that have been made worse by hormone therapy. Be careful, though. Too much DHEA—over 25 milligrams a day—can cause you to lose hair.

Since studies have shown that Tamoxifen can promote the growth of uterine and endometrial cancer, perhaps DHEA would be a more likely candidate to prevent breast cancer than a toxic agent that creates its own set of hazards.

In 1994, researchers at the University of California, San Diego School of Medicine wanted to find out what would happen to older individuals if they received DHEA supplements. The researchers gave middle-aged volunteers 50 mg of DHEA nightly for three months. The subjects reported enhanced energy, deeper sleep, improved mood, more relaxed feelings, and an improved ability to deal with stressful situations.

DHEA has been shown to help in the cases of dry skin, particularly common among women past menopause. Dry skin is a result of a drop in the production of sebum, an oily substance produced by special glands in the skin known as sebaceous glands. Sebum lubricates the skin. Dermatologist and researcher Dr. Norman Orentreich (the original developer of hair transplants) has shown that the functioning of the sebaceous glands is directly linked to DHEA levels. Our sebaceous glands produce huge quantities of sebum when our DHEA levels rise during puberty. (As a matter of fact, excess sebum can result in acne, a problem typical of adolescence.) Then, as our DHEA levels drop, sebum production falls off, and our skin gets drier. Dr. Orentreich has also shown that replenishing DHEA levels (via oral supplements or skin cream) can restore oil gland activity, returning sebum production to more youthful levels. The effect is to "plump up" the skin, giving it a more youthful appearance.

The body needs pregnenolone to produce adequate levels of progesterone, which in turn help balance estrogen levels and prevent problems such as cancer and fibroids associated with too much estrogen. It activates the immune system and is credited with enhancing memory and promoting vitality. Because of its ability to increase progesterone, it is a thyroid enhancer, helping the body produce enough thyroid hormone. This is very important, since the thyroid gland is the master hormone gland and regulates all the hormones. Anything that helps your thyroid produce hormones is going to help keep you healthy. The gland regulates growth and metabolism, and it releases hormones that affect numerous bodily functions such as heartbeat, temperature, digestion, calorie burning, and hair growth.

Pregnenolone is credited as being a potent memory enhancer. In one telling experiment, mice who were injected with pregnenolone retained their memories of a maze course taught to them by researchers, while mice who were not injected did not. Research on humans has shown improved hand-to-eye coordination, learning, memory, visual spatial tasks, and verbal recall.

Rahmawati Sih, M.D., Assistant Professor of Internal Medicine and Geriatrics at St. Louis University School of Medicine, became interested in pregnenolone while working with Dr. Morley on the mice experiment (mentioned above). In 1996, she conducted a brief study in which she administered a one-time dose of 10-500 mg of pregnenolone to humans to test the immediate effects on memory. Evidence shows the higher the dosage, the better the memory performance. No side effects were reported, and a few volunteers noted a decrease in their arthritis symptoms as well. In one study, depressed patients had lower levels of pregnenolone than healthy volunteers. Some doctors may find that pregnenolone's mood-elevating effects would reduce the need for antidepressant drugs.

Pregnenolone is synthesized in the body from cholesterol, and is produced both in the brain and the adrenal cortex. By the time we are 75, we are making 60 percent less pregnenolone than we did in our thirties. As our pregnenolone production drops, so does production of the other hormones.

Recommended dosages of pregnenolone, for men and women, range from 10 to 100 mg a day. Since hormones are complex, it is important to start low and slow. When DHEA first came out it was prescribed like popcorn. DHEA is best utilized in a trans-dermal cream form along with progesterone and pregnenolone.

The medical advances in the area of supplemental hormones are just beginning. Even as I write this, research is being conducted, products are being developed, and humans are being improved with the knowledge we have gained about hormones and how they work. Keep in touch with my work, and I promise to keep you informed about the fantastic advances to come.

8

*"A beautiful lady
is an accident of nature.
A beautiful old lady
is a work of art."*

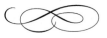

LOUIS NIZER

CHAPTER EIGHT

MIRROR, MIRROR

Liking What You See on the Outside

*If your face and body resemble the San Andreas
fault line with its cracks and fissures, don't despair!
Wrinkles can be reversed! If you have dry skin, and you're convinced
this fact of your nature puckers your pelt, think again.
To elude and eradicate your aging skin, you have to get under
your skin—where the problem really lies.*

THEY SAY TIME WILL TELL ALL. In the case of our faces, time may tell exactly how old we are or even imply we're older than we really are! But good nutrition and protection from the ravages of the elements can make time stand still or even go backwards to a less-wrinkled, more youthful appearance. In this chapter I will explain how. But first, a little lesson on what wrinkles are.

Imagine you've just bought a comforter. It feels soft and you enjoy running your hand over its smooth surface. Now imagine it's years later. The comforter has been washed dozens of times, rolled up, stored. . .you can get an idea of how it looks and feels now. The stuffing has lumps and bumps, and in some spots it has simply disappeared.

The collagen that gives structure to your dermis, or middle layer of skin, is just like the stuffing of that comforter. When your skin is in peak condition, its fibers are taut and elastic. Take care of it and it will remain pillow soft, smooth, and *wrinkle-free*. Abuse it, neglect it, ignore it, and the collagen fibers will become worn, thin, rough, and will hang loosely.

Joan Rivers was boarding a flight when she asked the stewardess where her seat was. "About three inches lower than last year," replied the stewardess.

Good nutrition and protection from the ravages of the elements can make time stand still or even go backwards to a more youthful appearance.

When we talk about treating wrinkles, we're really talking about taking care of the collagen and elastin fibers under the surface, in the dermis. If you look at progressive pictures of the face aging, you will see it is not wrinkles that age us as much as the transfer of fat downward. It's the combination of loose skin and a loss of fat that makes us look old. Over time fat disappears from the lips, the chin, around the mouth, the smile lines, temples, and the pads in the cheeks, which give you those youthful high cheekbones. When the fat is gone, the skin caves into wrinkles like the well-worn comforter.

We also lose bone structure. Osteoporosis starts in the bones of the head. This was validated for me when my slender, fine-boned shiatsu masseuse came to me moaning, "I have osteoporosis! What do I do?" By looking at her jaw I knew she hadn't heard the worst of it yet. The next day, dejected, she said, "I just saw my dentist. My gums and my teeth have disintegrated so badly I need $30,000 in dental work done."

Osteoporosis is most obvious when it affects the back bones, but it also reduces flattering high cheekbones and the prominent chin and jawline of a handsome man. Without proper nutrition to prevent bone loss, the elderly face is unrecognizable compared to its youthful counterpart. The section on osteoporosis in the chapter "Battles That Help You Win the War" will give you all the details to avoid bone loss. But in general you need to take your minerals, especially calcium, magnesium, and boron in solution, food sources of vitamin D and soy protein, which contain natural estrogen for hormone replacement. I take a supplement that includes green leafy vegetables for vitamin K. Natural progesterone cream is also recommended for postmenopausal women at risk for osteoporosis. Flavonoids, nutrients found in fruits and vegetables, combined with vitamin C, lay down youthifying layers of collagen, not just in the bones but also in the skin.

NEW OPTIONS FOR BEAUTY

For centuries people have established standards of beauty and altered themselves to reflect those standards. In some parts of Africa women aren't considered beautiful unless they wear lip plates.

Improving self-image is not the only reason we seek to make ourselves more beautiful. Over the centuries, people have made themselves more beautiful in order to: (1) acknowledge ourselves as human beings, (2) influence others, (3) outwardly communicate a more positive image, and (4) gain power and get material things.

People from all economic backgrounds have discovered that it is generally easier to get what you want from others if your looks are pleasing to the eye. Becoming more attractive is often a matter of necessity, not just aesthetics.

Another, less recognized benefit of the growth of plastic surgery in the U.S. are the philanthropic efforts of our surgeons. In poor countries, where surgeons are few or are inaccessible, U.S. doctors, such as Dr. Edward Terino and Dr. Angelo Capozzi, are donating their services so children, desperate for a life of normalcy and anonymity, can have their birth defects and physical abnormalities corrected. As U.S. clients demand better technology and techniques, Third World countries benefit from what surgeons learn in their practices.

In America we are extremely fortunate that beauty can be an option in our goal of personal growth; something we can choose rather than something we have to be born with. Options for outward beauty include jewelry, clothes, makeup, hairstyles and color, training in poise and grace, and, when more is desired, cosmetic surgery.

Cosmetic surgery in America used to be primarily for people with physical abnormalities. Thanks to a growing industry that has trained thousands of surgeons and that has realized incredible advances in technology, cosmetic surgery is available to anyone who can afford it.

As cosmetic surgeons went from repairing physical defects to restoring the youth of yesterday, many have lost the original premise of "plastic" surgery. The word *plastic* means "to mold or shape." Instead of molding or shaping the face into a more youthful look, they cut corners by simply pulling loose skin back over the face to stretch out the wrinkles, cutting off the excess. Cosmetic surgery is superficial, as is its outcome. Skin eventually loosens again, and the procedure has to be done over and over again.

The most common cosmetic surgery is the face-lift. The skin is loosened from the scalp and facial bones, and it is pulled upward to reduce sagging jowls, roofed eyelids, and highlight the cheekbones once again. However, if osteoporosis has reduced the cheekbones or jawline, the result is taut skin over a featureless face. The wrinkles may be gone, but so is the personality. A tight, lineless face is not youthful, it's skeletal.

Now there is a new breed of surgeons who are embracing the original goal of plastic surgery by molding and shaping the face to return the contours of youth.

Dermatologist Richard G. Glogau, M.D., San Francisco's preeminent doctor in the field of aging skin, says rejuvenation of the face involves more than just face-lifting, which redrapes the muscle and skin. To make the old face young, it must be filled out in the right places, giving back that fuller appearance. Dr. Glogau says, for a youthful look, replenish the fat. He masterfully takes fat from the other portions of the patient's body and moves it to the higher apples of the cheeks, which lifts the eyes and turns the corners of the mouth from a scowl to a smile. If you are considering a face-lift, the most common cosmetic procedure, Glogau says, "Tight is not right" and "Plump, not pull."

While you might consider such treatment, keep in mind there is a risk that you could be allergic if animal collagen is used. And surgical lifts are only a temporary solution. Eventually the sags and bags, lines and wrinkle furrows reappear as surely as a well-ironed garment gets creases.

Dr. Edward Terino, founder of the Plastic Surgeons Institute of Southern California, now in Thousand Oaks, is a pioneer in plastic surgery and leads the way with his latest techniques in three-dimensional facial contouring surgery using implants made out of a special material called "alloplastic." Using these implants, surgeons can augment skeletal deficiencies to achieve the firm contours, strong chin and jawline, and high cheekbones of youth. And in some cases, do away with the need for a face-lift.

Dr. Terino's talents as an innovator and scientist have produced a number of Terino implant designs that are available to surgeons and patients around the world. He has worked with scores of Hollywood stars to enhance their beauty. He shares Dr. Glogau's belief in "full, not pull" and his desire to educate his fellow surgeons make him a star attraction at symposiums and conventions. Dr. Terino has written a book, *The Art of Alloplastic Facial Contouring*, the most comprehensive source available on the subject of "plump, not pull" facial contouring.

Another pioneer in this new breed of surgical "sculptors" is Harry Mittelman, M.D., associate clinical professor of facial plastic surgery at Stanford University. He discovered that as we age we develop an indentation on the jaw between the chin and the jowl, which a face-lift cannot remedy. "About 20 percent of face-lift patients just need to fill in that groove area," says Mittelman. "The other 80 percent need the implant that adds structure to both the chin and jowl."

If you want to look into this option, make sure your surgeon specializes in facial contouring and has had extensive training in the use of facial implants.

Plastic surgery is an option, but it is expensive, and there are cheaper and less invasive alternatives. You can lift your face from the inside, providing your skin with the nourishment it requires to be as healthy as possible. Healthy skin is moist, smooth, glowing. In other words, young-looking skin.

NUTRITIONAL SOLUTIONS
TO SKIN PROBLEMS

For thousands of years humans lived mostly outdoors. No archeologist has ever reported finding anything even remotely resembling sunscreen along with the remains of primitive man. The sun has been around for millions of years, and only in our modern world have we been faced with skin cancer. Sunscreen use was rare in the 1920s, but the skin cancer rate was very low. Sunscreen use has risen every decade since then, and the rate of skin cancer has risen right along with it. Obviously it doesn't do a very good job of preventing skin cancer. So, if you want to prevent skin cancer, what do you do?

Here's how I manage to golf, play tennis, and ski without getting sun-dried leathery skin. I eat foods, use skin care products, and supplement with nutrients and natural ingredients that actually help protect and repair my skin from the ravages of the sun, elements and pollutants.

In previous chapters I mentioned the value of antioxidants in protecting the body against destruction by free radicals. We constantly need to be reminded of these specific nutrients that keep our bodies from breaking down, whether from injury, surgery, the sun, or time itself. They can mean the difference between a long-lasting infection and quick healing. Your antioxidant arsenal should include vitamin C with bioflavonoids, folic acid, vitamins A, B-12, and E, and selenium and zinc in a complete mineral formula in solution.

For faster healing, take at least 1,000 milligrams of bioflavonoid-enhanced vitamin C four times a day. Remember, it is the bioflavonoids that make all the difference. They hold up your skin cells just as chicken wire holds the wet cement of a wall under construction. Most cosmetic surgeons insist their patients quit smoking during recovery. Why? Because smoking restricts circulation in the skin. In contrast, vitamin E increases circulation.

We constantly need to be reminded of the specific nutrients that keep our bodies from breaking down.

Poor wound healing is one of the symptoms of scurvy, caused by a deficiency of vitamin C. A vitamin C deficiency can actually cause a breakdown of already healed wounds. Plasma vitamin C levels decrease during times of stress, bone fractures, burns, or major surgeries. Vitamin C, applied in lotion form on the skin, helps prevent skin damage from the sun's ultraviolet rays. If you use a lotion with vitamin C, make sure it includes the flavonoids. They diminish the effects of stretching and reduce puffiness.

In one study, the skin of live pigs was treated with topical vitamin C and then exposed to ultraviolet light at one to five times the dose that produces sunburn. The topical C not only protected the pigs from sunburn, but also protected the skin from cellular damage. The protective effect of the topical vitamin C lasted three days, even after the pigs were scrubbed with soap.

In a double-blind trial conducted at the University of Wisconsin at Madison, 48 out of 50 women felt that a cream containing vitamin C applied to the skin was more effective than a placebo—the fake stuff.

Researchers have noted that vitamin C acts as a sunscreen, and that its levels can be severely depleted after exposure to UV irradiation.

I have very sensitive skin that burns at the slightest exposure to sunlight. Reading these impressive studies, I wanted to test them. When I went skiing in the Austrian Alps (where high altitude intensifies the sun), I decided to take a major risk. I left my sunscreen in the hotel room and applied only a moisturizing lotion containing vitamins C, E, and B5.

I have to tell you, I was amazed! Not only did I not burn, after a full day of skiing in bright sunlight, but I actually tanned, probably for the first time in my life! What was most remarkable was that my skin didn't suffer any of the aging effects typically seen after exposure to the sun. What this meant for me was that for the first time my immune system was working to protect my skin. I am a believer!

Most people believe that oranges have the most vitamin C. They don't. In fact, black currants do. One orange contains approximately 70 milligrams of vitamin C, while a cup of black currants contains 202 milligrams. Other foods higher in vitamin C than oranges are papaya, guava, cantaloupe, strawberries, chili peppers, parsley, kohlrabi, broccoli, and kale.

Vitamin E has also been credited with reversing some of the effects of the sun. Undoing the damage caused by ultraviolet rays without a chemical face peel is almost impossible, yet, to some degree, vitamin E creams have helped certain individuals.

In tests conducted over a four-week period, 20 middle-aged women using a 5 percent vitamin E cream realized more than a 50 percent reduction in the length and depth of crow's-feet, those lines radiating outward from the eyes.

It is difficult to obtain extra vitamin E from foods. According to Orville A. Levander, from the USDA's Human Nutrition Research Center, Beltsville, Maryland, it is virtually impossible to obtain more than 25 International Units (IUs) of vitamin E per day solely from the diet. To protect the skin, the recommended dosage is 400 I.U. But to help things along, foods that contain vitamin E are wheat germ, seeds, nuts, oils, and cabbage.

A little-known but highly touted antioxidant is alpha lipoic acid. One of the things that happens as your skin ages is that free radicals break down the protein. Alpha lipoic acid is credited with stopping this process. In one study a topical form of lipoic acid helped prevent wrinkles and dry skin. Plastic surgeon Dr. Bruno Risto, of San Francisco, has his patients take it before, during, and after cosmetic surgery.

Your whole body, including the skin, can benefit from taking ALA orally (50-100 mg a day for a healthy adult is considered safe), as it has no known toxicity. Apply it topically in a cream containing at least 1 percent ALA prior to sun exposure. It boosts the skin's levels of glutathione, vitamin B6, and vitamin C to protect against sunburn and sun damage. Combine it with a cream containing vitamin C to increase the protective effects.

TAN WITHOUT THE BURN

I'm a California girl and in my youth spent 365 days a year in the sun, much to my grandmother's chagrin. I've always said one grandmother is worth three pediatricians. Mine used to admonish me: "Why are you spending so much time in the sun trying to look like a person of another race?" Like other girls of my generation we prized our tanned skin. But now we are paying the price in our later years. I wish I had known then about Dr. Meyer's work. You were smart enough to buy this book and read it, so you're ahead of me.

Over 50 years ago, before the advent of sunscreens, Dr. John Myers looked for a natural protocol to protect light skin from the aging and burning rays of the sun. People with fair skin— like mine—don't tan, we burn.

His protocol is especially important today for people who use tanning beds. Don't listen to what they tell you. Tanning beds have three times the harmful rays of the sun.

Dr. Myers reasoned that since the amino acid L-tyrosine is the precursor for skin pigment (melanin), nutrients that turn L-tyrosine into melanin would enable fair-skinned people to tan. Thousands of people have proven him right. And what are these nutrients? In the correct amounts, copper, vitamin B6, and vitamin C added to L-tyrosine result in a suntan in just two or three days.

Here's how it works. A few days before you plan to start, begin taking four milligrams of copper every day. Also supplement with 30 milligrams of zinc at the same time, since it nourishes the skin and balances the copper. Then take 1,000-1,500 milligrams of L-tyrosine, the same amount of vitamin C and 50 milligrams of vitamin B6.

Dr. Myers' protocol will not protect you against sunburn if you stay in the sun all day, but it will enable you to stay in the sun longer—in my own case 2½ hours. Continue to take precautions such as covering up, staying in the shade, and avoiding the most UV-intense times of the day: 11 A.M. to 3 P.M.

FATTY ACIDS—OILS FOR THE SKIN

Unsaturated fatty acids are required for all cell formation, including the cells that make up the skin. A deficiency of these nutrients may be responsible not only for dry skin but also brittle, lusterless hair, nail problems, dandruff, as well as eczema and acne. The best sources of unsaturated fatty acids, also known as essential fatty acids or EFAs (because your body cannot synthesize them and so they are essential to your diet) include the seed oils flax, pumpkin, soy, and walnut. Cod liver oil also contains an EFA. Keep in mind that EFAs are destroyed by heat, so if you think you're going to get them from fried foods, think again. The best way to eat these essential oils is with vinegar on salads. Try it! You'll be surprised how good walnut oil tastes in a nutty, fruity salad.

Borage oil is one source of essential fatty acids with such a reputation for benefitting the skin that the French put it in their skin-care products. My pets are all shelter animals. When I first took them in they were suffering from malnutrition and had the worst hair and dry skin you could imagine. I learned from experience that giving them borage oil and vitamin E turns their hair and skin to satin. We typically don't eat raw seeds and nuts, foods high in omega-6 essential fatty acid, which is why we need to supplement with it for healthy skin and hair.

Pantothenic acid, one of the B vitamins, is required for properly balancing fats and oils throughout the skin and is essential for proper skin function. Without it, the skin loses the ability to produce the sebum needed to moisten it. Sebum waterproofs and lubricates the skin. It's what makes your skin and hair feel a little bit greasy. Foods rich in pantothenic acid include brewer's yeast, legumes, whole grains, egg yolk, and salmon.

Vitamin B12 heightens and brightens skin color, helping to combat the discoloration of rosacea. Folic acid helps here too.

FOLIC ACID FOR SKIN REPAIR, DNA SYNTHESIS, AND CANCER PREVENTION

Despite its addition in "enriched" foods such as cereals and breads, folic acid still competes with essential fatty acids for the number one spot on the vitamin deficiency list, and since folic acid is destroyed by heat and sunlight, its destruction in skin exposed to ultraviolet light is what increases the risk of skin cancer. Folic acid, along with vitamin B6 and zinc, is absolutely key to DNA synthesis and repair in the skin, protecting the cells when they are damaged by sunlight.

I don't go anywhere without my supply of liquid folic acid. When I left it behind during a trip to France, I noticed the loss immediately. I was in Normandy, visiting the D-Day Memorial and Omaha and Utah beaches, retracing the battles famous for turning the tide of WWII. I was so overwhelmed with awe, emotion, and gratitude for the lives sacrificed that I lost track of time and came back to the hotel with a sunburn.

If you like to be out in the sun, have fair skin, and/or a family history of skin cancer, take at least one milligram (1,000 micrograms), or more, of folic acid daily. If you look at the amounts allowed by the FDA to be marketed in supplement form, it will seem like a lot. It's not. The FDA does not know how much folic acid is too much for the human body. And there have been no reported folic acid overdoses. The reality is that they don't know, so they force the consumer to take too little. This, despite countless studies that show higher amounts of folic acid are needed to maintain health and overcome disease. So, go ahead and take 1,500 micrograms. It won't be too much.

BEAUTIFUL, THICK, LUXURIOUS HAIR

At the same time proper nutrients are youthifying your skin, they can be giving you heavy, thick, gorgeous hair. Certain essential amino acids control the thinning and thickening of hair. Too little of the mineral magnesium, biotin, or inositol (B vitamins) can cause hair loss. Men shorted on folic acid sometimes become totally bald. However, in some instances, a normal intake of this vitamin restored their hair.

These are the key nutrients needed for normal hair growth: protein, magnesium, vitamin B6, folic acid, inositol, biotin, and PABA. Protein-packed foods include cheese, eggs, fish, soy flour, tofu, yeast, and yogurt. For megadoses of magnesium look to whole grains, green leafy vegetables, legumes, nuts, seeds, and shellfish. Foods fruitful in folic acid are torula yeast, brewer's yeast, alfalfa, endive, chickpeas, oats, lentils, beans, wheat germ, liver, split peas, whole wheat, barley, brown rice, asparagus, green peas, sunflower seeds, collard greens, spinach, hazelnuts, kale, peanuts, and fresh raw vegetables.

Beauty can be an option in our goal of personal growth—something we can choose rather than something we have to be born with.

Foods bountiful in B6 include brewer's yeast, blackstrap molasses, wheat germ, legumes, green leafy vegetables, and whole grains. Inositol-rich foods include whole grains, citrus fruits, brewer's yeast, blackstrap molasses, nuts, legumes, cabbage, and lecithin.

Biotin is abundant in egg yolks, unpolished rice, brewer's yeast, whole grains, and legumes. PABA-plentiful foods are sunflower seeds, brewer's yeast, and wheat germ. Only a small number of foods have been tested for PABA content.

Organic silica added to shampoo helps stop baldness, stimulates healthier new growth, and adds to the shine, luster, and strength of your hair.

Since amino acids are the building blocks of protein, adequate amounts are necessary for healthy hair. They include taurine, arginine, cysteine, acetyl-L-carnitine, and methionine. Large neutral amino acids are phenylalanine, leucine, isoleucine, tryptophan, valine, methionine, histidine, and tyrosine. They are essential to healthy communication between brain and muscles. Foods rich in these amino acids are as follows: Arginine: fish, poultry, and dairy products. Glutathione: raw green, yellow, and red vegetables. Canned or frozen vegetables lose glutathione during processing. Methionine: poultry, nuts, seeds, fruits, and vegetables. Tryptophan: turkey breast meat, wheat germ, granola, and oats. Tyrosine: peanuts, pickled herring, pumpkin seeds, and lima beans. Taurine: seafood, eggs, beans, and peas.

Even in her later years my mother had thick lustrous hair. She swears it was from bending over, every morning and night, to give her hair 100 brush strokes.

Gretchen, a great ski friend of mine was losing her hair in handfuls. I was baffled, as I had given her a solid regimen of minerals in solution, biotin, silica, B12, plus complete amino acids. It was on a four-day ski trip that I discovered she regularly took antihistamines for her allergies. The way antihistamines work is by shutting down blood vessels. Her restricted arteries were causing her to lose her hair. It was when she stopped taking the antihistamines that her body could take advantage of the nutrients, and her hair grew back.

ACNE AT ANY AGE

A study published in the October 1999 issue of the *Journal of the American Academy of Dermatology* found that of 749 adults between the ages of 25 and 58, 54 percent of women and 40 percent of men suffered from some form of acne. What's more, the prevalence of adult acne in both sexes did not decrease substantially until after the age of 44.

Whether you are a teenager afflicted with ongoing outbreaks, or a middle-aged woman pestered by premenstrual pimples, you can turn your pores to satin simply by taking zinc. I've seen hundreds of people who have tried, with little success, remedies from both over and behind the counter for their acne. Within months of starting a zinc regimen they cleared it up. The zinc treatment was first related to me by Dr. Robert Cathcart III.

Dr. Cathcart first learned of this pore-tightening acne antagonist from Dr. Michaelson of Sweden's Upsala University Hospital. Dr. Michaelson had prescribed 50 milligrams of elemental zinc three times a day with meals, and was astounded to note excellent results.

A renowned medical and alternative physician, Dr. Cathcart tried it on his patients and discovered that if the dosage were increased to 100-150 mg with each meal, patients got better results. He found that within 12 weeks, his patients taking the zinc improved their acne by a whopping 87 percent!

MINERAL RATIOS IMPORTANT

Minerals, among their many tasks (see previous chapters), are needed for the synthesis of enzymes. Enzymes run every operation in the cells and tissues of our body, including the renewal of skin, hair, and nails. They play a major role in the tone and elasticity of skin. The minerals of particular importance to the skin are selenium, which works with vitamin E to scavenge free radicals, and silica, which is a building block of collagen; and zinc, a co-factor with pantothenic acid in enzyme activity.

Researchers have found the calcium/magnesium ratio to be very important in maintaining the elastic quality of the skin. Dr. W. Muller and colleagues at the Institute of Pathology in Koln, Germany, examined the ligaments in the discs of spinal surgery patients, putting the patients into two groups: those with very elastic tissues, and those with non-elastic tissues. He found that among those with the most elasticity, a magnesium/calcium ratio in favor of magnesium was found.

This has been mentioned before but cannot be emphasized enough. Magnesium and calcium in combination work in balance throughout our bodies. Without magnesium, calcium accumulates in places it shouldn't. The consequences of taking calcium without magnesium is that calcium can crystallize, causing cross linkages. Many signs of aging then develop: arthritis, wrinkles, cataracts, and shriveled sex glands. Researchers call this aging process calcinosis. Calcinosis occurs because of a very common deficiency of magnesium.

You can give yourself a face-lift by providing your skin with the nourishment it requires to be as healthy as possible.

When we are born, our cells are 95 percent magnesium and 5 percent calcium. They are translucent. When we die, our cells are 95 percent calcium and 5 percent magnesium. Thanks to the crystallization of calcium, they are cloudy and inefficient. Making sure magnesium is always taken with calcium, and in solution, will prevent this sign of aging.

Copper and zinc are responsible for the expansion and contraction of cells, giving your skin youthful elasticity. Copper is noted as a nutrient important to the manufacture of elastin in the skin. It acts as a catalyst, forming certain enzymes involved in the cross-linking of collagen and elastin. On the face, symptoms of a copper deficiency include sallow, puffy skin, uneven skin tone, and patches of red irritation. Studies have shown when copper is low, changes occur in connective tissue and the skin begins to sag, especially the buttocks and cheeks. One way to gauge your biological age is to pinch the skin on the back of your hand and see how long it takes to spring back. The faster it returns, the better your elasticity.

Make certain to get your minerals in a solution form. The way nature ushers us out of the world is to cut back on our ability to absorb nutrients. Minerals are essentially metals, and they are extremely difficult for the body to absorb in tablet form. The body must break down a hard tablet to solution. A mineral already in solution helps rejuvenate the body by delivering these hard-to-process, vital beauty-enhancing elements to the cells.

ACID THAT MOISTURIZES

Studies have made a connection between wrinkle formation and something called hyaluronic acid, or sodium hyaluronate, a naturally occurring skin and tissue lubricator found in certain skin care products. Wrinkles and a loss of elastin are believed to be caused by free radical damage. Recently, another factor has been considered inadequate: the aforementioned hyaluronic acid.

Researchers never fully realized the connection between hyaluronic acid and skin until they reviewed the results of a breakthrough study on sheep fetuses. Scientists were looking for substances that would repair wounds without scar tissue or damage to the elastin. They began to study fetal lambs because of their ability to heal without scar formation. They discovered fetal wounds contain high levels of hyaluronic acid. They also discovered high levels of hyaluronic acid in the amniotic fluid—thus it continually bathes the fetus and encourages smooth cell formation.

A Basil, Switzerland, pharmaceutical company credits hyaluronic acid with not only moisturizing the skin, but "helping to maintain or restore the biophysical properties of skin, such as smoothness, elasticity, and resilience, which gives it its youthfully fresh appearance."

An article in the *International Journal of Dermatology* reported on a study that linked a lack of sufficient hyaluronic acid in the skin to wrinkles and skin sags (loss of elastin), which are typical of advancing age. I was so impressed with this and the other studies I researched that I formulated a skin care product for my own use, containing hyaluronic acid, the previously discussed vitamin supplementation, and certain skin care foods, e.g., cucumber.

BEAUTIFYING BOTANICALS

Certain foods have been shown to be helpful for skin healing and fortifying. Cucumber is one of them. For centuries, cucumber has been used as a toner after cleansing, and as a bleaching agent in freckle creams. A cucumber's natural acidity is close to that of normal skin. This makes it non-irritating and helpful in restoring the skin's acid balance after cleansing.

In the 17th Century, in his book *Complete Herbal*, herbalist Nicholas Culpeper said of cucumbers: "The face being washed with their juice cleanseth the skin…" and "cureth the reddest face that is; it is excellent, good for sunburning, freckles and morphew." Morphew is an obsolete name for a condition that results in dry, scaly skin.

American pioneer women rubbed cut cucumber over their sun-battered skin to soothe and smooth. What's good for the pioneer is good for the modern-day woman. For a quick cool-off pluck a cuke from the fridge, cut off a chunk, remove any seeds (a minor inconvenience), and rub the cut side all over your face, neck, and shoulders. Let the juice dry.

Once in Las Vegas, since I don't drink or gamble, I did the next most harmful thing. I lay in the sun until I turned a blistering red. I called room service for an order of cucumbers, rubbed them all over my stinging skin, and experienced instant and blessed relief.

There's also some evidence cucumber soothes inflamed tissues. Cucumber contains vitamin C (a component of collagen) and chlorophyll, said to be useful in wound healing.

Because of its numerous beneficial properties and its clean fragrance, cucumber juice is used in many creams and lotions, soaps, sunburn preparations, masks and packs, wrinkle treatments, and bleaching aids.

For softer skin slab on a little papaya, also rich in vitamin C and bioflavonoids. It contains papain and the digestive enzyme tyrosine, a natural meat tenderizer that helps remove the protein deposits that contribute to stiff, hard skin.

The skin care products I helped formulate, use, and recommend contain extracts of lime tree, birch bark, geranium, rosemary, sandalwood, clove, and marigold, also called calendula, which helps heal dry skin. Oak bark contains large amounts of tannin, which acts as an astringent, in that it closes pores and stimulates blood circulation. It helps prevent red, rough irritated skin. Sage is another herbal that acts as an astringent. It is a component of some medicines for mouth and throat afflictions.

Geranium oil is a superb addition to any skin care line. I find that it refreshes, invigorates, and clears my skin, combating oily, congested complexions or inflammations. It can help with acne breakouts, and it helps prevent the minor infections that make blemishes worse.

Chamomile is also found in many skin medications. In folk medicine, it has been used to treat inflammation (applied externally as a poultice in the early stages). Ointments containing chamomile or extracts of chamomile have been used for the prevention and treatment of cracked nipples and diaper rash.

I also like to use glycyrrhizinic acid, a licorice extract, because it helps to reduce the inflammation of irritated skin, and is so potent that it is used to treat peptic ulcers. I retard age spots with licorice root. I was convinced to use it by reviewing the results of laboratory experiments that demonstrated how licorice root reduces the activity of the cells responsible for age spots.

Around the world researchers are hard at work analyzing the many medicinal properties of the approximately 600 varieties of aloe plants. Refined aloe, the gel-like pulp of the plant, is being used successfully to treat burns, x-ray and radiation dermatitis, gastric ulcers, sunburn, frostbite, gastrointestinal disorders, constipation, sports injuries, diabetes, etc. I include it as a therapeutic ingredient for my skin. I've proven to myself that aloe penetrates injured tissue, relieves pain, has anti-inflammatory properties, and dilates capillaries, thereby increasing circulation.

A 1993 Japanese study of the application of witch hazel (*Hamamelis virginiana L.* bark extract) determined it is helpful in preventing wrinkles. It was also found to be a potent scavenger of free radicals. In lieu of an alcohol-based toner (which dries the skin) after washing my face thoroughly, I use witch hazel with chamomile, aloe vera gel, cucumber and licorice extracts, and allantoin. This formula speeds up the production of epithelial cells, i.e., those that fill in and heal wounds, like the craters formed after a pimple erupts.

SOLUTIONS TO COMMON PROBLEMS

Certain topics come up every time I discuss aging. Age spots and skin tags are age-related annoyances that can be eliminated.

What causes age spots? Scientists believe they are caused by accumulations of lipofuscin in the skin, a fatty substance that attracts pigment. Retinitis pigmentosa, an age-associated eye problem, is also believed to be caused by lipofuscin accumulations. What is interesting is the number of studies that show vitamin E can reverse this accumulation. In humans, lipofuscin is reportedly associated with liver and intestinal diseases, which impair vitamin E absorption and utilization. In animals it is found when they are vitamin E deficient. A deficiency of vitamin A has also been associated with lipofuscin accumulation.

They're annoying, some think ugly, but they are generally harmless. They are those pinches of skin that seem to serve no purpose or have a reason to exist. Laypeople call them skin tags. Doctors call them acrochordon or cutaneous (skin) papillomas. Put away those scissors, skin tags can be prevented by eliminating sugar. Skin tags are a direct result of an imbalance of glucose. Start by eating foods low in sugar—the low glycemic foods outlined in the weight loss chapter—and eliminating processed food from your diet. Include anything that contains corn syrup. Adopt a whole-food diet with no refined sugar, flour or caffeine. Take a supplement formula that includes folic acid, the B vitamins, C, E, and a mineral in solution formula that contains chromium. Chromium is important to regulating blood sugar.

REJUVENATING SKIN WITH NATURAL ACIDS

Researchers have discovered that alpha hydroxy acid (AHA), found in apples, grapes, and other fruit, can help to remove shallow wrinkles and rejuvenate the skin. It removes dry skin, scaly patches, age or brown spots, and acne, as well as wrinkles. I first wrote about AHA in my 1988 book, *Foods That Heal*, and I have been using it ever since. Here's a recipe for alpha hydroxy cream. Cook a cored and peeled apple in a little milk. Mash the apple in the milk. Cool the mixture. Then apply it once weekly and leave it on the face for 15 to 30 minutes.

Smiling, even or especially when you're down, calms your whole nervous system, lightens your mood, and brightens your looks.

Alpha hydroxy acid is a collective term for the various acids found in certain fruits. AHAs are actually citric acid, glycolic acid, lactic acid, malic acid, and tartaric acid.

Ladies of the court of Louis XIV are said to have applied old wine to their faces to remove wrinkles and blemishes. Old wine contains large amounts of malic and tartaric acid.

Polynesians, who get lots of tropical sunlight, replete with skin-damaging ultraviolet radiation, use a mixture of citrus and sugar cane juice to keep their skin healthy. These foods contain citric and glycolic acid.

Cleopatra indulged in milk baths and yogurt facials. Sour milk and yogurt contain substantial amounts of lactic acid, which is an effective skin moisturizer and also helps skin shed its outer layer of dead cells more easily. The ancient Egyptians, believing their pharaohs and queens to be gods, invented special milk baths and shampoos to keep their hair and skin looking appropriately "God"-like.

FORTIFYING THE SKIN

Collagen is the stuffing in your body. When it's in peak condition its fibers are taut and elastic. Take care of it and the surface will remain pillow soft and smooth. Throw it around, squeeze it and abuse it, and you'll see the results. The collagen fibers will become worn, thin, rough, and hang loosely.

Collagen needs certain nutrients to grow and stay healthy. Scientists have found that collagen is largely made up of silica. So what do you think nourishes it the most? Silica!

Formulas that contain silica have proven effective in the prevention and repair of stretch marks. In one controlled study, researchers found an average 70 percent prevention rate and a 15 percent success rate in diminishing existing marks.

Silica is also important to healthy nails. If yours are dark, brittle, and have an abnormal surface, they deserve a closer look. It could be that a deficiency of silica is robbing the calcium from your body and you haven't noticed—yet.

A friend of mine swears by aloe vera and vitamin E. Look for the combination in skin lotions. Smear it all over every morning and evening—and don't wait until you see evidence of expansion. Not only are you treating the skin for the stretching, but you're conditioning it to withstand it.

FACIAL WORKOUTS

Lift that chin, stretch that brow. Facial exercises can tone and tighten the face the way that calisthenics firm the body.

FOR MOUTH-TO-CHIN FURROWS:
1. Lift the lower lip into a "pout."
2. Pucker lower lip, bringing both corners toward the center;
3. Relax the lip. Repeat ten times.

FOR FROWN LINES:
1. While looking straight into a mirror, try to bring your eyebrows to the center of your face.
2. Lift eyebrows as high as possible. Repeat five times.

FOR DOUBLE CHIN:
1. Lie on bed with your head hanging over.
2. Slowly open your mouth.
3. Slowly close your mouth. Repeat opening and closing mouth ten times.

A healthy blood flow carries oxygen and nutrients to all the cells of the body, including the skin. Here are several ways to increase that flow. Tilt feet up on a slant board for 15 minutes every day, massaging the face and scalp to reverse the effect of gravity and bring blood and nutrient supply to skin, hair, and eyes. Your eyesight diminishes in direct relationship to blood supply to the eyes. Regular, aerobic exercise stimulates blood flow to the muscle tissue. Simply applying fingertip pressure to lines on the forehead, under the eyes, and sides of the mouth can help circulation.

Jack LaLanne offers this tip for firming a double chin. While sitting in a chair, extend your jaw in an exaggerated chewing motion that stretches the muscles under the chin and front part of the neck. Another exercise for sagging jowls and loose cheeks is to clench your teeth and stretch your lips as far as possible into a grimace. Then say "aaargh" through the corner of your lips (which sums up how I feel about droop and sag, in general).

Best exercise: Put on a happy face. Smiling, even or especially when you're down, calms your whole nervous system, lightens your mood, and brightens your looks. Even if you have to put a pencil in your mouth and force yourself. Your subconscious will catch up with your face and say, "Hey, this person is happy. We'd better get in step here."

9

"No diet will remove
all the fat from your body
because the brain is entirely fat.
Without a brain you might
look good, but all you could do
is run for public office."

COVERT BAILEY

CHAPTER NINE

MAUREEN'S WEIGH-LESS AGE-LESS DIET

Common Sense Principles of Weight Gain and Loss

After an exhaustive multi-million-dollar health study, the government concluded that people would live longer if they didn't die sooner.

I WILL TELL YOU POINT BLANK — YOU CAN ACCEPT IT WITHOUT QUESTION. A key to longevity is diet. How you eat influences your health and your figure. I do not espouse the virtues of one diet over another. Biological individuality dictates we are too different from one another to have one perfect diet apply to all.

Currently, the blood type diet is a biggie. It assumes that people of the same blood type have consistently the same propensity for weight gain. The only thing consistently in evidence is that when people eat a primitive diet they stay slim and healthy. When they move to the typical "Western" diet, they get fat. There are few obese people in Ethiopia, no matter what their blood type.

There are hundreds of diet books and articles on weight loss. I can't possibly anticipate each of your individual tastes, habits, and lifestyles. What I *will* do is lay ruin to those myths that say the longer you live, the more pounds you put on; and demonstrate to each of you how a combination of eating well (wisely), nutritional supplementation, and easy exercise will keep you toned, trim, and, most importantly, **healthy**. No matter how thin you are, if you aren't healthy, you won't look good. My goal here is to provide you with the tools and information needed to make you proud of who you are and what you see in the mirror each and every day.

YEARS DO NOT EQUAL FAT

Some of us may be guilty of being mean-spirited when observing how some people have aged. Remember when Marlon Brando was the movie industry's sex symbol? Remember when Mickey Rooney was a heel-kicking, energetic star of stage and screen?

If you've let yourself put on the pounds as you counted off the years, you might be secretly pleased to see how they've aged, and, wrongly, feel better about yourself as a result. With all that money and power, if they couldn't do it, how can I expect to?

Because you care, and you want to be a better person, or you wouldn't be reading this book. If you've read this far, you've learned about many successful agers. The people who look and feel great in spite of, or because of their years. You are never too old to learn—do you mind hearing that again?

The long-held belief that body fat increases as people age is challenged by a study published in the *Journal of the American Geriatrics Society*.

The study evaluated 679 people from 29 to 94 years old. The researchers concluded that the increased body fat often seen in older adults results from weight gain rather than an inevitable change in body composition with age. In fact, Dr. Andrew Silver, at St. Louis University School of Medicine, found no significant increase in the percentage of body fat after the age of 40.

In some cultures, such as the natives of the South Sea Islands, the old are as slim as the young. They are also just as active and childlike. So if you're using aging as your excuse, drop it. You can no longer blame your birthdays for your weight problem.

A key to longevity is diet. How you eat influences your health and your figure.

I once went to an exclusive little gym run by a 75-year-old matriarch. I was doing something wrong on one of the machines and she hit me! Although I certainly don't advocate violence, I appreciated her feistiness. Have you ever noticed how the most crotchety, angry, irritating people are often the most successful? They are also the thinnest. If you can have the energy to be irritated, and expect perfection of yourself, you can lose weight and keep it off.

Energy is a wondrous thing. But it's elusive and deceptive. You think you don't have it, but you do! The fact is, the more you exercise, the more energy you have. Then you want to exercise more, and you actually miss it if you don't. Less exercise means less muscle and more fat.

Over time, fat, especially in the face, moves downward, creating pockets under the eyes, sagging jowls and less plump to the cheekbones. The puffy soft look that is a sign of a sedentary lifestyle is not youthful or attractive.

Around the body, fat falls to the underside of the upper arms and the back, and the buttocks become uneven. As the skin thins, the underlying cellulite fat becomes more noticeable. It is not the weight we gain that contributes to our aging appearance, it's where the associated fat we add ends up. Lose the fat and you may lose some of that aging look.

Look at movie stars as they age. They don't all undergo cosmetic surgery. Many have rigorous exercise and diet regimens that keep them looking young. Gloria Swanson looked youthful at 84. She wore diaphanous dresses that showed a washboard stomach. Thin and gaunt is neither attractive or youthful. It's not thinness that is ageless, it's a strong slimness. Consider Tina Turner. She's not thin by any stretch of the imagination. But she looks terrific. She's strong and healthy, and she looks good.

With a healthy diet, you can be proud of who you are and what you see in the mirror each and every day.

Weight loss begins and ends with the mind. There is a close correlation between the craving center of the brain and the eye. See it once and you are tempted—the second time you are lost. That is why so many restaurants display desserts in revolving, lighted cases. The first time you see it you are tempted. The second time you are lost. Everyone has the potential to gain too much weight. Even me.

I was recently a guest lecturer on a cruise to Portugal and had to host tables at dinner. They say the appetite comes with the food.

I had to watch people eat Austrian pastries—the kind my grandmother used to make. My old addiction for sweets crept up on me, like a monster waiting in the cellar to be freed and devour my willpower, and I could not resist joining them for dessert. I gained weight. I had conquered my sugar cravings for years before I went on the Portugal cruise. I took great joy and satisfaction in this accomplishment.

I didn't need or desire sweets, but like a dragon living in the basement waiting for me to open the trap door, I came back from my working vacation once again addicted to sweets. It took a resolve of the mind, then putting my resolve into action by arranging my environment to again overcome my addiction and lose the weight I had gained. How did I do this?

I eliminated all high caloric food: bread, butter, cheese, desserts, starchy sweet fruit, and milk products. The most difficult part for me is avoiding the myriad of temptations presented at restaurants, supermarkets, bakeries, and dinner parties. What were some of the techniques I used to avoid temptation? They were as follows:

1. Rid the kitchen of offending foods (you know where you store those tempting betrayers). Your first line of defense is not having "danger" foods in the house (they don't appear on their own).

2. Divert your eyes from sweets that are, by the way, intentionally placed at eye level at the grocery store checkout stand, and don't shop while hungry.

3. Make a shopping list, and stick to it. Bring only enough money to pay for what you need.

4. No wandering into the middle of the store where the dead foods are. Stick to the outer aisles where the live foods are (life comes from life).

5. When you are tempted by a white or brown "unfood," visualize it as white or brown death. Then rid yourself of the thought. Don't let it take root in your mind.

6. As you experience a craving, consider it a good thing and learn to enjoy it. Let denial be your friend—making you svelte, vibrant, and vigorous. Don't consider it a deprivation.

7. Stop and ask yourself if you are eating because you are hungry, or are you eating for face entertainment? If you are not hungry, don't eat. This is why most diets work at first. They make people more conscious of what they eat, how much, and if they are really

hungry. Make those hunger pangs your criteria for eating.

8. The subconscious doesn't register a negative: "No, I can't have dessert." Rather, consider yourself full. If you're at a dinner party, politely decline your hostess's offering while diverting your eyes from the dessert.

9. Compliment the hostess and the love and time she poured into the delicious food and eat a small portion. Don't leave uneaten portions on your plate in front of you. Call the food server or take it away from your range of vision.

10. Eat slowly to convince your body it is being satisfied. Chew your food 20-30 times per bite. For assistance, eat to slow music. You'll chew in direct rhythm with the music you're listening to. Mozart wrote table music. You'll eat less and enjoy it more if you give your body the time to tell you that you are satisfied.

11. And, most importantly, I never eat after 7 P.M. I told this to a friend of mine who wanted to lose weight. When I saw him six months later I was astounded. He had lost 60 pounds! He said all he did was stop eating anything after 6 P.M. every night.

Weight loss is still a matter of eating less and exercising more. Eat dinner as early as you can or not at all. Go for a walk instead. Substitute eating a large dinner with going to the gym. Take a walk. Eating before going to bed or those midnight raids in the kitchen are a ticket to weight gain. Not eating late in the day is a good way to take off the pounds. Your meals should be low fat, low calorie, and small portions. Eat no more than you can hold in your two cupped hands at one time.

For dinner, try eating a salad with raspberry vinegar. Here's a recipe (included in my book *The Light at the End of the Refrigerator*) for an excellent raspberry vinaigrette: two tbsp. raspberry vinegar, ½ cup olive oil, ⅛ tsp. black pepper, ⅛ tsp. white pepper, ⅛ tsp. nutmeg, four cloves garlic, chopped, and several mint leaves, crushed. Sometimes I add a pinch of cayenne pepper for punch.

I've traveled the world and discovered cultures that eat small amounts of highly nutritious food are the people who are the healthiest and leanest, and live not only longer, but better. While in Africa, I lived with the Masai, a joyous people who laugh easily and continuously. They only eat once a day, and only as much as they are able to hold in their two cupped hands, the size of your stomach.

A combination of eating well, nutritional supplementation, and easy exercise will keep you toned, trim, and, most importantly, healthy.

The Masai are lean and muscular, as if they were carved out of ebony. From them I learned that less food means more energy. I saw them eat the smallest meals with the least calories, and they could still run miles without stopping—laughing the entire way. The whole six weeks I was in the Africa bush country I saw only lean, healthy people.

The first fat Masai I encountered was when I went into the city of Nairobi. She was leaning against an ice cream stand, eating an ice cream cone. The Masai I lived with didn't have ice cream, and it shocked me when I realized how accustomed I'd become to their appearance.

I recently spent time in Bermuda, Portugal, and France. In those countries the people walk everywhere, and they eat wholesome meals devoid of the chemicals, transfats, and processed starches we consume daily. Their agricultural techniques include letting the soil lie fallow so it may remineralize and support the foods grown on it with optimum nutrition. I saw few obese people.

But when my plane landed in the Los Angeles airport, there

they were. A 1994 JAMA study reported that three out of every ten adults is obese. Looking around that airport, I would have guessed the rate to be a lot higher. We know more about diet and nutrition than any country in the world, but we currently bear the distinction of being the fattest nation in today's world, and in the history of the world.

CONQUERING OUR CRAVINGS

Did you know that 90 percent of people with Type 2 diabetes are obese? Type 2 diabetes occurs when glucose cannot enter body cells. Sometimes called "adult onset diabetes," it is typically diagnosed among middle-aged, overweight, inactive people. The same things found to help Type 2 diabetics also help lose weight and restore health.

Type 1 occurs when the pancreas loses its ability to produce insulin, for whatever reason. It used to be called juvenile diabetes because it is commonly diagnosed in childhood.

Regulating blood sugar is very important to weight loss. If you're prone to cravings, you are probably addicted to sugar. Eating too much sugar is more than the three tablespoons you put in your coffee or the daily candy bar. Most processed foods contain a lot of sugar and corn syrup, and certain fats common in processed foods increase the body's production of sugar. Too much sugar in the diet is known to cause Type 2 diabetes.

Beware the insidious corn syrup. It's in everything from ketchup to canned beans. One of the reasons we like the taste of processed food is because of their high levels of salt and sugar. Our tastebuds have become accustomed to the sugar in our food, and without it they are unhappy.

Also, beware of diet drinks and candy, especially those with aspartame, or Nutrasweet. Aspartame is a chemical, and a potentially dangerous one at that. Better to get used to the taste of iced tea without sugar than to use the chemicals in that blue packet to sweeten it. Aspartame has been linked to diabetes, blindness and other eye problems, brain tumors, joint pain, and even multiple sclerosis. What they aren't telling you is that when you put a case of soda in your garage or car trunk, and it gets hot, the chemical sweetener breaks down into formaldehyde—that's the liquid that preserves body parts and dead animals. If you had to dissect frogs in school, you took them out of jars of formaldehyde.

The Department of Health and Human Services lists more than 100 symptoms attributed to aspartame, including difficulty breathing, vomiting, and headaches.

Problems are so common that there is an Aspartame Victims Support Group for those who found out too late and want to help others discover why they are sick with no diagnoses available. Their website is full of revealing facts, studies, and testimonials. Want to know more? Their website address is http://www.presidiotex.com/aspartame/index.html.

Americans drink, on average, 41 gallons of soda per year. Soft drinks have diuretic properties and increase water losses, threatening dehydration and its subsequent problems. For every soda you drink, you should consume one glass of water.

Whole civilizations, previously exempt from diabetes, once introduced to affluence and the accompanying Western diet (high in saturated and transfatty fats and sugar), have found themselves in an epidemic of diabetes and obesity.

Today's modern diet is replete with unhealthy transfatty and saturated fats. Fat in the bloodstream blocks the effectiveness of insulin, making the body believe it needs to convert more muscle to fat. What portion of our weight-related issues are a direct result of insulin problems? It is probably a very high percentage.

What is it about our modern-day diet that contributes to obesity and diabetes? Demineralized foods, sugar, and inactivity.

Leviticus 26:26: "…and ye shall eat, and not be satisfied."

More than 99 percent of the U.S. population is deficient in trace minerals, according to U.S. Government document #249. According to U.S. Senate document #264, our farm and range soils have been depleted of nutritional minerals with the result being that crops grown on these soils are mineral-deficient.

A U.S. Department of Agriculture study done at Tufts University, Boston, found that 85 percent of the American public is deficient in one or more of the nutrients for which recommended daily allowances (RDAs—I call them recommended deficiency allowances) have been established.

A deficiency of certain minerals has been linked to blood sugar regulation and an inability to lose weight.

CHROMIUM AND VANADIUM FOR BLOOD SUGAR BALANCE AND FAT LOSS

There is a reason why so many people are feeling tired and putting on excess weight. It's the same reason that too many people develop heart disease or diabetes: most people are deficient in essential trace minerals, including chromium. A chromium deficiency causes fatigue, excess fat production, and can be a major contributor to heart disease and diabetes.

To lose weight you must eat less calories, more nutritious foods, and exercise more.

Chromium is a mineral used to treat low blood sugar. As a co-factor to insulin, chromium is central to the body's utilization of blood sugar, and studies have shown it helps eliminate or reduce the insulin requirements of diabetics.

Chromium may assist in weight loss because high blood levels of insulin, which occur as a consequence of tissues' resistance to insulin, promote excessive deposition of fat. Chromium reduces insulin resistance, which in turn decreases our storage of body fat and increases its metabolism. Since chromium helps stabilize blood sugar levels, it also may reduce the feeling of hunger.

Chromium may help suppress the appetite because both chromium and insulin stimulate serotonin, a brain chemical important to feelings of well-being and satisfaction. A deficiency of serotonin has been linked to depression.

Vanadium, a little-known mineral, works with chromium and is important in regulating blood sugar. It regulates cholesterol levels, helping to prevent circulation blockages. Because of its glucose-regulating qualities, it can help battle fatigue, depression, and nervous exhaustion. It is found in safflower, olive and sunflower oils, whole grains, herring, sardines, and liver.

These minerals are vitally important to your health, yet dangerously rare in the modern diet. They are more likely to be in short supply than other minerals, and are, perhaps, the missing link in the incredible epidemic of obese and overweight Americans. I say this because studies have demonstrated that when they are supplemented weight loss is very common. They are only part of the equation. To lose weight you must eat less calories, more nutritious foods, and exercise more.

THE GLYCEMIC INDEX

If you could eat certain foods you knew helped you lose weight, would you? Of course you would. A newly discovered food principle, essential to any discussion of weight loss, involves how fast or slow a particular food digests, and the amount of blood sugar—or glucose—is released as a result. I've already discussed the concept of blood sugar levels effecting weight loss. The story continues.

Carbohydrate foods that break down quickly during digestion have the highest glycemic indexes. High glycemic foods—

potatoes and white bread—digest quickly, make the body crave more, and keep blood sugar levels high. Overweight and obese people typically have high blood sugar levels.

Carbohydrates that break down slowly, releasing glucose gradually in the bloodstream, have low glycemic index values. Examples are corn, oatmeal, whole grains, and lentils. It is the low glycemic foods that satisfy hunger without high calories and are important to any program of weight loss.

The difference between high and low glycemic foods is the amount of fat they contain. Low glycemic foods are low in fat and calories. Choose lean meats, high grain breads, whole grain cereals, lowfat milk, yogurt, vegetables, and fruit. But eat carbohydrates like grains with your fruit and vegetables. Avoid anything fried, such as french fries and potato chips. Skip the margarine, fatty cheese, and fatty meat.

Maximum Living Nutrition Bites are a natural, nutritionally complete meal replacement product.

There is a food you can accurately call a diet food. It is vinegar. As little as four teaspoons of vinegar in a vinaigrette dressing, taken with an average meal, lowers blood sugar by as much as 30 percent, plus it stimulates hydrochloric acid in the stomach, the digestive juices needed to break down food. Among the various types of vinegar, red wine is the best. Also, lemon juice has been found to be advantageous.

With improved digestion and absorption, the body stores less fat. Along these lines, I must stress the importance of digestive enzymes. The proteolytic enzymes, especially, are important to digesting and assimilating protein so it isn't stored as fat. For the fat you eat, enteric-coated enzymes, that aren't digested in the stomach, will help your body break it down so it isn't stored in the tissues.

BURNING FAT WITH APPETITE-CONTROLLING CARBOHYDRATES

Complex carbohydrates such as brown rice, beans, lentils, or whole grain bread not only are digested slowly, thus stabilizing blood sugar, but their high fiber content helps control the appetite and increase energy.

Do you crave sweets in the morning and fats for lunch? Make a habit out of eating things like lentils, kidney, navy, or pinto beans for breakfast. For lunch, have a salad with vinegar and olive oil and maybe some whole grain bread drizzled with olive oil. Make sure that whatever food you eat, it is whole, raw, and contains its natural fiber.

Beans are great for weight loss and regulating blood sugar because their natural sugars are burned off slowly, thereby stabilizing blood glucose and acting as an appetite suppressant. Beans also contain B vitamins, which are important to the nervous system, brain function, and energy level.

The best way to lose weight and keep it off is to convert fat into muscle. You need to burn 3,500 calories in order to lose a pound of fat. As you lose fat and gain muscle you speed up the weight loss process. Pound for pound, muscle burns five times as many calories as other body tissues. The addition of ten pounds of muscle to the body can burn 600 calories more a day. That means after the first three months or so you can cut down and take it easy without seeing the pounds come back. You also need adequate amounts of water and the nutrients that make up muscle: amino acids, (the end product of protein digestion), minerals, and essential fatty acids.

There is a natural, nutritionally complete meal replacement product I am very excited about. I love the taste and smooth, chewy consistency. It's called "Maximum Living Nutrition Bites, the feel-full snack." It nourishes muscle, helps burn the fat, and restores the body to optimum health. I've tried it, and it works for me. It is packaged as chewy nuggets and comes in three flavors: chocolate, vanilla nut, and peanut butter.

Its main ingredient is soy protein, a healthy, easily digested protein that helps convert fat into muscle. The soy protein in these tasty snacks also contains many other vital nutrients, including fat-reducing enzymes, nitrogen, and amino acids.

Centuries of making people both healthy and slim has proven what a health-giving food soy is. It is rich in soluble and insoluble fiber, and contains the good fats (monounsaturated and polyunsaturated fats, and omega-3 fatty acids), which help the body move out the bad lumpy fat. Not only does soy contain *no* cholesterol, but it is also known for its ability to remove it from the body. Soy also provides all eight of the essential amino acids not manufactured by the body, and isoflavonoids, which act as natural non-steroidal estrogen. Soybeans, a fabulous cancer fighter, are eaten in great quantities in Japan and China, and is one of the reasons researchers believe these countries have low rates of breast cancer and few menopausal symptoms.

Maximum Living Nutrition Bites have all of the good stuff and none of the bad stuff. They have all the nutrients necessary to lose weight and build lean muscle: essential fatty acids, amino acids, minerals, and soy protein. Unlike most products like it, they contain no hydrogenated oils or refined sugar. The following fat burning ingredients are in them: biotin, because it helps eliminate the body's need for glucose, increasing the body's ability to burn fat and reversing the unhealthy aspects of being overweight; chromium for blood sugar regulation, an important factor in weight loss; lecithin and the minerals zinc and copper, so as the pounds roll off, your skin will stay tight, firm, and beautiful; and digestive enzymes that speed up weight loss by encouraging thorough digestion so nothing is left to be stored as fat.

Amino acids are included because they are needed to convert fat to muscle. The amino acid carnitine is particularly helpful, as it is well-known and well-researched for its ability to burn fat, especially when exercising. Glutamine, another amino acid, is included to help the nerves cope with the stress of dieting.

Maximum Living Nutrition Bites also include natural, not synthetic, tryptophan, an all-important amino acid that manufactures serotonin in the brain. Serotonin helps the hunger center of the brain do its job. Maximum Living Nutrition Bites are high in appetite-suppressing fiber—at least two grams per serving—and zero cholesterol. Because this soy product so encourages lean muscle, my personal trainer, Chris Mullen (everyone should have a Chris), recommends taking it every 2½ hours through the course of the day so you sustain and increase fat-burning lean muscle mass.

I lost ten pounds after my gluttonous cruise trip with his help. I lifted weights (and supplemented with the other nutrients that manufacture lean muscle mass in the body—amino acids, minerals, and essential fatty acids like borage oil and flaxseed oil), and I drank at least a gallon (eight glasses) a day of purified water. Even though Maximum Living Nutrition Bites contain vitamins and minerals, I still take my minerals in solution twice a day, along with my nutritional regimen.

Protein is important for converting fat into muscle. In fact, all food contains some amount of protein. Eat protein early in the day, while the body is physically active. If you want a nice piece of salmon, have it for breakfast or lunch.

Protein doesn't have to come from one source and doesn't have to be eaten for dinner. If you don't care for fish, eggs, chicken, or meat to reach your daily allowance of complete protein, try combining small amounts of whole grains with legumes. Remember, eat only what your two cupped hands will hold.

The Greek dish falafel combines whole wheat pita bread

with garbanzo beans. It happens to be a healthy, fast, finger food, and makes a delicious meal. Latin Americans get their protein by combining corn tortillas with beans. In India it's rice or wheat chapatis with lentils. Because cooking can destroy many essential amino acids, try to avoid processed foods and eat your veggies raw.

Amino acids are also important to regulate mood and overcome depression and are responsible for some of the emotional reasons we crave food. The brain uses amino acids to produce its most powerful mood-elevating chemicals: serotonin, dopamine, endorphin, and gamma-amino-butyric acid (GABA), which is naturally more relaxing than Valium. Supplementing with a complete amino acid formula will help stabilize your brain chemistry, lower your appetite, elevate your mood, and overcome your desire for unhealthy comfort foods. Try to take your amino acids at least 20 minutes before or 20 minutes after a meal in which you eat protein, otherwise the protein in your food will compete with the amino acids and some will not get to the brain.

How do you eat less without lowering your fat-burning ability?

By eating less food gradually, so your system adapts, making sure what you eat is high in nutrients, complex carbohydrates, and low in fat. We can accomplish this goal by grazing, i.e., eating small meals every two to three hours. Maximum Living Nutrition Bites are ideal for this purpose, and you don't have to cook!

According to Susan Smith Jones, Ph.D. (health sciences), a fitness instructor at UCLA, "grazing" will virtually prevent carbohydrates and proteins from being converted into fat. Like adding more wood to the fire, eating small meals, or snacking on Maximum Living Nutrition Bites, will keep the metabolism burning the fat.

The typical dieter skips meals, especially breakfast. This is the worst meal to exclude. It is the equivalent of a fast, sending the wrong message to the body. You may skip breakfast because you are not hungry. If you skipped dinner, you would be hungry. If you eat a heavy meal for dinner, your body has to work overtime digesting it. There is a reason most fatal heart attacks occur in the early hours of the morning. The body uses a tremendous amount of energy digesting food while resting. This is very stressful on the heart, stomach, and all the other organs.

If you're going to skip a meal, make it dinner. It's obviously healthier, and you sleep better when you're not digesting food. Not only that, but growth hormone, (which diminishes as we get older and may be the reason we look older and get fatter) increases with good sleep on an empty stomach. If you are going to eat dinner, make it a salad with my raspberry vinaigrette dressing. Vinegar increases digestion, and the fiber in lettuce, an old folk remedy for insomnia, helps you sleep.

THE TRUTH ABOUT SOY

As with nutrients and anything else, there is nothing so uncommon as common sense. When someone tries to put down a food, eaten by millions of people for centuries, not only without harm, but with benefits such as lower incidences of breast cancer, menopausal symptoms, and heart disease, I always question their biased point of view. Especially as they ignore 300,000 deaths a year from doctor-prescribed drugs.

Without benefit of cited research, one misinformed author makes a bold claim that soy products are "quite dangerous."

In a Harvard Medical School newsletter, *Women's Health Watch* (August 2001), an article entitled, "What we still don't know about soy," states that, "Soybeans are unique among plant foods in supplying all the essential amino acids that the human body needs, making soy protein similar in quality to meat protein—

but with largely unsaturated instead of saturated fat. In addition, soy contains the isoflavones genistein and daidzein, plant hormones that seem able to either mimic or counter the effects of estrogen. They have been proposed as helpful in preventing several hormone-related diseases."

Even people who should know better, rather than looking into the studies themselves, repeat misinformation, conjecture, and thin-ice research that, when examined, proves to be less than convincing.

When you come across claims that soy is problematic, it is important that you evaluate the source of the information. The person making the claims should cite studies to back them up. But don't stop there. Look at the title of the article, consider how long ago the study was conducted, and the source of the information.

One diet book states that "despite all the fanfare about soy being a miracle food for menopausal women, there are actually no documented benefits from soy phytoestrogens for menopausal women." This misinformed author wasn't looking very hard.

The Harvard newsletter article states that soy products are associated with fewer hot flashes and, "Because soy isoflavones have certain estrogenic effects, women and researchers have looked to soy as a possible alternative to standard hormone replacement therapy."

The Harvard article also cites a study showing an increase in bone mineral content and density after postmenopausal women took an isoflavone-rich soy preparation.

Of course, it's important to realize soy is no magic pill. Alleviating menopausal symptoms and osteoporosis requires weight-bearing exercise, a healthy diet rich in fruits and vegetables, and supplemental vitamins and minerals. For more on solutions to menopause and osteoporosis, read the chapter in this book "Battles That Help You Win the War."

Another published claim was that "Soy's estrogenic effects are associated with elevated rates of breast cancer." This author's claim was based on a study of women with "estrogen receptor-positive" cells. This means they were already sensitive to estrogen. It's like giving milk to someone who is lactose intolerant, then proclaiming milk to be harmful to everyone. Even if this were true, historically we'd see more incidences of breast cancer among Japanese women over many decades. In reality we don't.

In an article published by the North American Menopause Society in their July-August, 2000 issue ("The Role of Isoflavones on Menopausal Health"), the authors summarize much convincing research to refute this common allegation.

"In vivo, high concentrations of the isoflavone genistein inhibit most types of cancer cells... In a case-control study, a significant reduction in breast cancer risk was seen among premenopausal and postmenopausal women," and "In a study of Asian-Americans, increased tofu consumption was significantly associated with decreased breast cancer risk."

An article in *Nutrition Cancer* ("Dietary Antioxidants During Cancer Chemotherapy: Impact on Chemotherapeutic Effectiveness and Development of Side Effects," Conklin KA, Nutr Cancer, 2000;37(1):1-18) states that genistein has anti-estrogenic properties and that it **inhibits the growth of human breast cancer cells in culture.**

The Harvard newsletter states that, "Soy isoflavones resemble tamoxifen...already used for breast cancer prevention. Isoflavones also have anti-tumor activity and block the formation of blood vessels in chemically induced breast tumors in animals," and "When premenopausal women drink isoflavone-containing soy milk, it significantly lowers their circulating levels of both estrogen and progesterone, potentially protecting them from estrogen's cell-stimulating effects."

One of the most nefarious claims is, "Infants of both sexes who are fed soy milk **MAY** later develop hormonal abnormalities such as early menstruation or delayed male genital development."

The fact is, infant formulas are notoriously deficient in minerals and essential fatty acids, vital to the growth of the infant. Notice the word "may." This indicates the cause and effect is not certain. If it's not certain, why bring it up at all?

In one six-month study on osteoporosis, postmenopausal women showed an increase in bone mineral content and density in their lumbar spine after taking an isoflavone-rich soy preparation. Rather than highlight this truth, the authors of the study chose to emphasize the fact that there was no increase in the thigh bone. Reporting on this study, Harvard researchers admitted that had the scientists continued the study over an extended period of time, they would likely have seen better results. Six months is too short a time-frame to see results in studies of food products.

THE PARADE OF DIETS

Searching the Internet under the term "weight loss," I found 1,130 books available on a bookstore website. This demonstrates the public's serious need and desire to find answers to weight loss.

The good news is that as we become more educated and aware of nutrition, many of these books emphasize healthy, nutritional eating.

The bad news is marketing ploys and fraudulent claims are still rampant. If it's so simple, as one book title says, why do you need "1001 Ways"? Other titles promise "30 Days to Swimsuit Lean," or "32-Days to a 32-Inch Waist." This can only be true if you began with a 26-inch waist.

Beware of claims that promise you'll "Lose weight quickly and easily." If I lost substantial weight in 30 days, I'd assume I was sick. Fast weight loss is a symptom of disease. It's not natural and it's not healthy. Your body needs to lose weight gradually so your organs can keep pace.

Beware of diets that depend on one food or nutrient.

Dr. Atkins' massive marketing firm says to eliminate whole grains. They are a vital source of B vitamins, important to clear thought and good mental health. Then he advocates high protein, which has been associated with breast cancer and ovarian cysts. A high protein diet uses up your proteolytic enzymes (the ones that digest protein), so there's not enough left to keep cancer in check.

At the other end of the spectrum is Dean Ornish's plan, which discourages fat and protein. Protein is essential for muscle production. If you exercise, you need protein to convert fat into muscle.

We are indebted to Dean Ornish for his profound studies on reversing heart disease with diet, but many find his diet is too hard to follow. Furthermore, he has yet to see the light on nutritional supplementation. He's too principled to turn a blind eye to the plethora of scientific studies on the use of supplementation in weight loss and wellness.

Our bodies are composed of a cornucopia of nutrients and chemicals, and we must address those elements in our diets. Our varied nutritional requirements must be met or we get sick and die.

Beware of diets that omit anything, including fats. Even saturated fat, in small amounts, is necessary for health, and some fats are so nutritionally advantageous—and commonly missing in our diets—that we should be seeking them out. I'm talking about the monounsaturated and polyunsaturated fats, and omega-6 fatty acids found in nuts and certain vegetables. In addition, our bodies need the omega-3 oils found in fish and flaxseeds.

A deficiency of fatty acids has been linked to cravings for fatty foods. When we aren't getting enough good fats, our body tells us to eat the bad.

What is important, when evaluating diets, is to use common sense. Realize that nothing works exactly the same for everyone. If certain supplements or foods "feel" wrong, or produce undesirable symptoms, omit them. Also, no matter how "good" the food might taste, you could be allergic to it.

By using common sense, moderation, and intelligence, and by listening to your body, you will find the diet that's right for you and watch those pounds melt off.

CAUSES OF WEIGHT GAIN

If your weight fluctuates, especially if you feel heavier at the end of the day, consider the possibility that you have food allergies. Food allergies can cause women and men to retain water and, thus, weight. When the body reacts to an allergen it naturally swells. If, when you wake up in the morning your tongue has small tooth-shaped wedges grooved into the side of it, chances are you have food allergies. There is a simple, scientific test you can peform to identify your food allergens in my book *All Your Health Questions Answered Naturally.*

Identifying and eliminating food allergens can stop this cycle. Common food allergens are beef, sugar, dairy, chocolate, eggs, citrus fruits, coffee, corn, malt, pork, potatoes, tomatoes, wheat, and yeast.

An inability to lose weight can also be caused by an under-functioning thyroid, called hypothyroidism. When the thyroid is under-functioning, the metabolism slows and it can become difficult to lose weight.

The late Broda O. Barnes, M.D., Ph.D., was a world-renowned thyroid authority. He concluded that first generation hypothyroids often can correct their condition by taking a kelp tablet daily. Kelp is rich in iodine, the thyroid's major nutrient. Hypothyroids of the second generation or beyond can overcome depression and many other symptoms of low thyroid function by taking a natural, desiccated thyroid supplement prescribed by a physician.

Dr. Barnes' best contribution toward public awareness of thyroid problems was in all likelihood the Barnes Basal Temperature Test. This is a simple test that can be done by anyone in the privacy of his own home.

Since your body temperature reflects your metabolic rate (which is largely determined by hormones secreted by the thyroid gland), the state of the gland can be determined by taking your temperature. All that is needed is a thermometer.

Shake down the thermometer and place it by your bed before going to sleep. When you wake up, prior to getting out of bed, place the thermometer under your armpit for a full ten minutes. Stay as still as possible. After ten minutes, read and record the temperature and the date. Record the temperature for at least three mornings, preferably at the same time. Menstruating women should perform the test on the second, third, and fourth days of menstruation.

Your basal body temperature should be between 97.6 degrees F and 98.2 degrees F. Anything lower may indicate hypothyroidism. Anything higher may indicate hyperthyroidism.

Hormones are a problem when it comes to weight loss. For two years, I've been working with two women on their weight. While they have both adjusted their eating habits, neither has lost fat. I've recently learned that they're both on synthetic hormones. As much as 35 pounds of their weight is a side effect of the hormones.

Candida Albicans, or yeast infection, has been associated with weight gain and is often caused by chronic use of antibiotics. It can be fought with supplemental beneficial bacteria, e.g.: lactobacillus acidophilus, which is found in yogurt and other cultured food. Liquid garlic extract has also been found to be helpful. I would also abstain from sugar entirely, even fruit, for a few weeks.

Another cause of weight gain is toxins stored in body fat. According to Hans Kugler, Ph.D., an authority on health and aging, for both anti-aging and weight loss purposes, we need to eliminate the toxic chemicals in our bodies.

It is very simple. Take a non-flushing niacin (a B vitamin). There are several types you can buy in a health food store, such as nicotinamide or niacinamide hexanicotinate. These are non-flushing niacins. For detoxification, an hour to an hour and a half before sweating take about two grams of a non-flushing niacin. Induce sweating, either by exercising strenuously or by sitting in a sauna.

The more you exercise, the more energy you have.

Antioxidants with good quality essential fatty acids, such as borage oil and flaxseed oil, activate lipids (the fat turnover) and the toxic chemicals that sit in the adipose tissue and the nerve cells. If you do this about three times a week, you can remove approximately 66 percent or two-thirds of the toxic chemicals in your body in around four weeks' time. According to Kugler, along with the chemicals, you can also expect to lose five to 15 pounds of weight.

There is a precaution you must consider with the use of niacin. High doses of niacin, especially the non-flushing forms, are highly effective for removing cholesterol but can cause liver inflammation. While taking niacin have your natural healing doctor periodically run a blood test called "liver enzymes." If the test shows your liver has become inflamed, all you need to do is stop taking niacin and the problem will rapidly disappear. However, you should avoid high-dose niacin entirely if you already have liver problems or consume a lot of alcohol. Also, don't take niacin if you are on cholesterol-lowering drugs or herbal supplement formulas designed to lower cholesterol.

EXERCISE BURNS FAT

"Food fuels the furnace of metabolism; exercise stokes its fire."
MAJID ALI, M.D.

You've heard the term "feel the burn"? Exercise instructors use it to describe the burning sensation resulting from strenuous exercise. If your idea of vigorous exercise is eating faster, join the Rockettes. You don't have to bounce and bobble your way to a good figure; rather, you can experience burn by simply lifting your leg repeatedly. This simple exercise will burn fat and build muscle.

To achieve fat-burning in exercise merely requires slow, sustained activity. Forty-five to 60 minutes of vigorous walking is recommended, every day if possible.

I love dancing. My friend Owen Meldy, a life-long dancer and instructor, emphasizes the social nature of dancing. Dancing, any kind of dancing, is a thrill, as well as a pleasurable form of exercise. "When you dance, every part of you comes alive; mind, body, and spirit," he says.

Dancing is the perfect way to alleviate the boredom and self-punishment we sometimes associate with exercise. It's more than just moving your feet. It's also moving your heart. In addition to the physical benefits that energize your whole being, every cell of your body is flooded with an infusion of life-affirming joy, and every pore of your skin expels the toxins created by stress and boredom.

During our Portugal cruise, Meldy taught us a fascinating new dance called Universal Swing. It was so much fun that I easily danced off several pounds of those pastries. You don't have to leave the floor with Universal Swing because the steps he teaches can be adapted to everything but a waltz. (If you'd like to learn more about Universal Swing, you can check out his website at www.universalswingdance.com or e-mail him at owen@universalswingdance.com.)

Want to feel the burn? Try this. Hold your arm out, palm upward. Now lift it up. Do it twice. No problem, right? Now, do it twenty times. Did you feel the burn? Now do it while holding a can of soup. Better yet, my book, *All Your Health Questions Answered Naturally*. You just increased the burn by including something heavy. This is called weight- or resistance-training.

You can burn fat while watching TV. From your couch or chair, lift your legs twenty times. Next add ankle weights. Now you're doing weight-training. This form of exercise not only burns fat but increases muscle. If you keep adding weight, you'll keep adding muscle (more so for men, but women can do it too). As you gradually add weight (or resistance), you add strength. If you keep it up, you can compete with body-builders. And it doesn't matter how old you are—even if you're 95 you can do it!

As I mentioned before, building muscle through regular strength training enables you to burn more calories every single day—even while you are resting. One pound of muscle burns 35 to 50 calories a day. Compare that to a paltry two calories burned by a pound of fat.

Have you seen those photos of muscle-bound women who didn't stop until every last morsel of fat was converted to muscle? Fat flees their bodies like Superman is repelled by Kryptonite. Even their breasts have been converted! There's nothing left! This is an extreme I don't agree with. But you can see for yourself how this works and, to a much lesser degree, make it work for you.

As you walk to exercise your legs and lower body, carry weights and swing your arms to burn off the fat in your arms and upper body.

Orchestra conductors have notoriously strong arms and cardiovascular health because of the repetitive motion their profession requires. Swimming is good for burning fat because of the resistance provided by water. Most classes begin with water exercises (to increase stamina) before getting out there to sprint and tread water for 30 minutes at a time. For the less ambitious, water aerobics offers resistance with less work, and it's great for cardiovascular fitness.

TEN STEPS TO WEIGHT LOSS

1. ***Exercise every day.*** Walk one day, take an aerobic class the next, lift weights the next. Take dance classes. Join a dance club. Vary your exercise to keep you interested. If you join a Universal Swing Dance class, you'll feel like Ginger Rogers or Fred Astaire in two classes and look like them in six. (Remember, www.universalswingdance.com.)

2. ***Skip dinner if possible, or have a light salad and exercise before bed.*** Don't eat for two, ideally three, hours before bedtime. Studies on human growth hormones show they not only encourage a thin physique, but are increased when you sleep on an empty stomach. Other ways to increase growth hormone is to exercise and get a good sleep.

3. ***Eat no sugar and no more than two servings of fruit a day.*** Eliminate high sugar fruits like mango, peaches, and bananas, and target apples, grapes, and watermelon.

4. *Avoid processed grains.* This means white bread, white or instant rices, and dry pasta. All your grains should be whole, not processed. Limit your bread consumption to whole grains and only two pieces a day.

5. *Eat protein food only at breakfast or lunch.* Have lentils, kidney beans, navy beans, or pinto beans for breakfast. For dinner, have a salad with my special raspberry vinaigrette. To keep the body's fat burning oven stoked continuously, snack on a product like the Maximum Living Nutrition Bites.

6. *For between-meal snacks eat lean foods or two Maximum Living Nutrition Bites nuggets.* Target foods such as carrots, broccoli, plain popcorn, or whole grain crackers. Eat an apple chewed slowly with a large glass of water.

7. *Eat no dairy products, including cheese, for the first three weeks.* Because weight gain is associated with food allergies, and because dairy products are common allergens, staying off dairy products for a few weeks might tell you how much they are to blame. Get your calcium from a mineral drink that contains a 3-to-1 ratio of magnesium to calcium in solution.

8. *Supplement with a multi-mineral formula in solution that contains chromium, vanadium, and biotin.* You'll notice you experience cravings during certain times of the day. Pay attention to when your cravings occur, and take the mineral in solution formula half an hour before they happen.

9. *When dining out, if there are portions left on the plate, leave or have the plate taken away.* Don't look at it. Remember, your stomach is the size of your two hands cupped together. Try to limit your intake to the amount your

hands will hold. This formula has served me well especially because I have small hands. When your hostess is ladling out portions at a dinner party, tell them the story about the Masai of Africa. It makes great dinner conversation.

10. **Drink lots and lots of water.** Drink at least eight glasses or two gallons a day. Nothing makes you lose excess fluid like drinking a lot of water, so it's good for losing water weight.

Remember, you didn't put on those extra pounds overnight. Therefore, you must realize that those pounds are not going to come off in a couple of days. You must have patience, perseverance, be disciplined, and understand that to lose the weight and keep it off you must be willing to make permanent changes in your approach to eating and exercise. Malcom Forbes said it best, "Diamonds are just chunks of coal that stuck with it."

Most importantly, never lose sight of your goal, and remember that good health and longevity are your primary objectives.

Remember, God rewards faithfulness. The fact that you, as well as your family, friends, and business associates, may consider you more attractive and you will have a more energetic and confident approach to life are tremendous, but merely "secondary" benefits. Vibrant good health is its own reward.

REFERENCES

A

Adams, Ruth, "Versatile Vitamin E," *Better Nutrition for Today's Living*, v. 53, n. 4, p. 14, April 1991.

Adler, T., "Alzheimer's Causes Unique Cell Death," *Science News*, v. 146, p. 198, September 24, 1994.

Adler, Nancy; Matthews, Karen, "Health Psychology: Why Do Some People Get Sick and Some Stay Well?" *Annual Review of Psychology*, v. 45, p. 229, Annual 1994.

Adlercreutz, Herman, et al., "Plasma Concentrations of Phyto-Estrogens in Japanese Men," *The Lancet*, v. 342, November 13, 1993.

Aero, Rita; Rick, Stephanie. *Vitamin Power*, New York: Harmony Books, pp. 39, 63, 72-73, 81, November 1988.

Allison, Malorye, "Stopping the Brain Drain," *Harvard Health Letter*, v. 16, p. 6, October 1991.

Ames, Bruce N., "Dietary Carcinogens and Anticarcinogens; Oxygen Radicals and Degenerative Diseases," *Science*, v. 221, p. 1256, September 23, 1983.

Anderson, Richard A., "Chromium, Diabetes Mellitus, and Lipid Metabolism," *Journal of the American College of Nutrition*, v. 11, n. 5, October 1992.

"Anti-Aging News," *Longevity*, p. 8, January 1994.

"Antioxidants May Protect Our Eyes," *Better Nutrition for Today's Living*, v. 53, n. 9, p. 10, September 1991.

Appleton, Nancy, *Lick the Sugar Habit*, Garden City Park, New York: Avery Publishing Group, 1988.

Ask-Upmark, "Prostatitis and Its Treatment," *Acta Med. Scand.*, v. 181, 1967.

B

Balazs, Endre A.; Denlinger, Janet L. "Viscosupplementation: A New Concept in the Treatment of Osteoarthritis," *The Journal of Rheumatology*, v. 20, Supplement 39, pp. 3-8, 1993.

Barinaga, Marcia, "How Long Is the Human Life-Span?" *Science*, v. 254, n. 5034, p. 936, November 15, 1991.

Berger, Stuart, *Forever Young—20 Years Younger in 20 Weeks*, p. 206, Avon Books, New York, 1989.

Besdine, Richard W.; Singer, Karl, "Successful Aging for All?" *Patient Care*, v. 28, n. 4, p. 7, February 28, 1994.

"Beyond Vitamins," *Newsweek*, April 25, 1994

Binkley, N. C.; Suttie, J. W., "Vitamin K Nutrition and Osteoporosis," *Journal of Nutrition*, v. 125, pp. 1812-1821, 1995.

Blakeslee, Sandra, "The Return of the Mind," *American Health: Fitness of Body and Mind*, v. 8, p. 94, March 1989.

Bland, Jeffrey S., "Back to Basics: Dietary Fiber, Perimenopause and Estrogen," *Let's Live*, April 1995.

Bland, Jeffrey S., "How Young Are You? Good Habits, Nutrition & Antioxidants Can Slow Down Biological Aging," *Health News & Review*, v. 3, n. 2, p. A, Spring 1993.

Block, Gladys, "Vitamin C and Cancer Prevention, The Epidemiologic Evidence, *American Journal of Clinical Nutrition*, January 1991.

Boers, G.H.J., "Hyperhomocysteinemia: A Newly Recognized Risk Factor For Vascular Disease," *Netherlands Journal of Medicine*, v. 45, p. 34, 1994.

Borokhov, David Zakharovich, "Education Level and Length of Life of Kazakhstan Town Residents," *Sotsiologicheskie Issledovaniya*, v. 17, n. 9, pp. 98-101, 1990.

Bortz, William M., II, "Geriatrics: The Effect of Time in Medicine," *The Western Journal of Medicine*, v. 166, n. 5, p. 313, May 1997.

Bracki, Marie A.; Thibault, Jane M.; Netting, F. Ellen; Ellor, James W., "Principles of "Integrating Spiritual Assessment into Counseling with Older Adults," *Generations*, v. 14, n. 4, p. 55, Fall 1990.

Brand-Miller, Jennie; Wolever, Thomas; Colagiuri, Stephen; Foster-Powell, Kaye, *The Glucose Revolution*, Marlowe & Company, New York, 1999.

Brattstrom, L. E., et al., "Folic Acid Responsive Postmenopausal Homocysteinemia," *Metabolism*, v. 34, pp. 1073-1077, 1985.

"Breast-Feeding Boon to Infants in Third World," *Medical Tribune*, v. 11, October 3, 1991.

Brown, Katrina M., et al., "Vitamin E Supplementation Suppresses Indexes of Lipid Peroxidation and Platelet Counts in Blood of Smokers and Nonsmokers but Plasma Lipoprotein Concentrations Remain Unchanged," *American Journal of Clinical Nutrition*, v. 60, p. 383, 1994.

Brownlee, Shannon, "Blitzing the Defense; Piercing the Brain's Protective Barrier Is Key to "Treating Many Serious Neurological Disorders," *U.S. News & World Report*, v. 109, n. 15, p. 90, October 15, 1990.

Bruckheim, Allan H., "House Call: Yes, There Are New Recommended Daily Requirements," *The Kansas City Star*, October 31, 1994.

Bulcroft. Kris; O'Conner-Roden, Margaret, "Never Too Late," *Psychology Today*, v. 20, p. 66, June 4, 1986.

Burton Goldberg Group, *Alternative Medicine, The Definitive Guide*, Future Medicine Publishing, Inc., Puyallup, Wash., 1993.

C

Caffery, Barbara E., "Influence of Diet on Tear Function," *Optometry and Vision Science*, v. 68, n. 158-72, 1991.

Canty, David J.; M.S., Zeisel, H, M.D., Ph.D., "Lecithin and Choline in Human Health and Disease," *Nutrition Reviews*, University of North Carolina at Chapel Hill, Chapel Hill, NC, 27599-7000, U.S.A., p. 52, October 1994.

Cardozo, Constance, "Mind Spas," *Harper's Bazaar*, v. 125, p. 140, February 1992.

Carlier, C., et al., "A Randomized Controlled Trial to Test Equivalence Between Retinyl Palmitate and Beta Carotene for Vitamin A Deficiency," *British Medical Journal*, v. 307, pp. 1106-1110, 1993.

Casson, Peter R., M.D., et al., "Oral Dehydroepiandrosterone in Physiologic Doses Modulates Immune Function in Postmenopausal Women," *American Journal of Obstetrical Gynecology*, December 1993.

Challem, Jack, "Breast Cancer: Tracing Its Elusive Causes and Leveraging Dietary Strategies to Prevent It," *Let's Live*, p. 19, November 1994.

Charaskin, E., *Vitamin C—Who Needs It?* Arlington Press & Company, p. 151, 1993.

Chopra, Deepak, *Ageless Body, Timeless Mind*, p. 193, Harmony Books, 1993.

"Chromium-Rich Barley Effective Treatment for Diabetes," *The Nutrition Report*, March, v. 10, n. 3, 1992.

Cichoke, Anthony J., "Sports Injuries," *Better Nutrition*, v. 62, n. 1, p. 20, January 2000.

Clare Ansberry, "Bonne Bell Retires Stereotypes," *The Wall Street Journal*, February 5, 2001.

Clark, Linda, M.A., *A Handbook of Natural Remedies for Common Ailments*, Old Greenwich,

Conn.: The Devin-Adair Company, pp. 55-59, October 1976.

Clarkson, Thomas B., et al., "Estrogenic Soybean, Isoflavones and Chronic Disease Risk and Benefits," *Trends in Endocrinology and Metabolism*, v. 6, 1995.

Cohen, L.; Kitzes, R., "Infrared Spectroscopy and Magnesium Content of Bone Mineral in Osteoporotic Women," *Isr J Med Sci*, v. 17, pp. 1123-1125, 1981.

———. "A Total Dietary Program Emphasizing Magnesium Instead of Calcium," *Journal of Reproductive Medicine*, v. 35, pp. 503-507, 1990.

Constantinidis, Jean, "Treatment of Alzheimer's Disease by Zinc Compounds," *Drug Development Research*, v. 27, p. 12, 1992.

"Copper and Its Possible Role in Cardiomyopathies," *The Nutrition Report*, v. 89, p. 96, December 1993.

Cowan, L.D., et al., "Breast Cancer Incidence in Women with a History of Progesterone Deficiency," *American Journal of Epidemiology*, v. 114, pp. 209-217, 1981.

Culbert, Michael L., D.Sc., "Live Cell Therapy: A Time Honored Modality and an Important Part of 21st Century Medicine," International Health and Education, Inc., San Diego, Calif., 2000.

———., "Live Cell Therapy: Medicine for the New Millennium," International Health and Education, Inc., San Diego, Calf., 2000.

D

Darby, Robert D., *Telomere Cancer Theory*, darby@hctc.com, 1977-2000.

Darrach, Brad, "The War on Aging," *Life*, v. 15, n. 10, p. 32, October 1992.

Davidson, Jacqueline, "Longevity Blooms with Younger Grooms: Research Shows that Women Married to Younger Men Live Longer than Expected," *Psychology Today*, v. 23, n. 12, p. 72, December 1989.

de Vries, Jan, *Life Without Arthritis*, London: Mainstream Publishing, pp. 24-25, 30, 1991.

Delaney, Lisa, "Awaken the Doctor Within!" *Prevention*, v. 45, n. 10, p. 58, October 1993.

Dossey, Larry, M.D., "Beyond the Body: Prayer's Health Powers," *Fitness*, pp. 114-115, May/June 1994.

Dreher, Henry, "Why Did the People of Roseto Live So Long?" *Natural Health*, v. 23, n. 5, p. 72, September/October, 1993.

Dunne, Lavon J.; Kirschmann, John D., *Nutrition Almanac*, Fourth Edition, MacGraw-Hill, 1996.

———., *Nutrition Almanac*, Third Edition, McGraw-Hill Publishing Company, 1990.

Dychtwald, Ken, "Toward a New Image of Aging," *Prevention*, v. 42, p. 103, June 1990.

E

Earl, William L., "Relaxation Groups and the Aging: Suggestions for Longevity," *Nursing Homes*, v. 36, n. 16, September/October 1987.

Editorial, "Breast Cancer, Have We Lost Our Way?" *The Lancet*, v. 341, n. 8841, p. 343, February 6, 1993.

Ehrenreich, Barbara, "The Change: Women, Aging and the Menopause," *Time*, v. 140, p. 80, October 26, 1992.

Elias, Marilyn, "Mind and Menopause," *Harvard Health Letter*, v. 19, November 1993.

Elin, R., "Magnesium: The Forgotten Nutrient," *The Nutrition Report*, February 1995.

Erasmus, Udo, *Fats and Oils*, Alive Books, Burnaby, B.C., Canada, 1986.

Erickson, Deborah, "Human Growth Hormone Could be a Blockbuster," *Scientific American*, v. 263, p. 164, September 1990.

Evans, Gary, W., "The Effect of Chromium Picolinate on Insulin Controlled Parameters in Humans," *International Journal of Biosocial and Medical Research*, v. 11, n. 2, 1989.

Evans, Imogen, "The Challenge of Breast Cancer," *The Lancet*, v. 343, n. 8905, p. 1085, April 30, 1994.

"Expectation of Life in Years," New York Public Library and The Stonesong Press, Inc., 1993.

F

Faelton, Sharon, *The Complete Book of Minerals for Health*, Rodale Books, Emmaus, Pa., p. 427, 1981.

Fahim, W. S., et al., "Effect of Panax Ginseng on Testosterone Level and Prostate in Male Rats," *Arch. Androl.*, 1982.

Falsini, Benedetto, "Spacial-Frequency-Dependent Changes in the Human Pattern of Electroretinogram After Acute Acetyl-L-Carnitine Administration," *Graefe's Archives Clin. Exp. Ophthalmol.*, v. 229, pp. 262-266, 1991.

Feinblatt, H. M.; Gant, J.C. "Palliative Treatment of Benign Prostatic Hypertrophy: Value of Glycine, Alanine, Glutamic Acid Combination," *Journal of the Maine Medical Association*, 1958.

Felter, H. W., M.D., *The Eclectic Materia Medica, Pharmacology and Therapeutics*, Eclectic Medical Publications, Portland, Oreg., 1983.

Findlay, Steven, et al., "Iron and Your Heart," *U.S. News & World Report*, v. 113, n. 11, pp. 61-67, September 21, 1992.

Fink, Joseph M.; Edelson, Richard L., "The Immunologic Function of Skin, *Scientific American*, v. 252, p. 46, June 1985.

Fischer, Joan; Johnson, Mary Ann, "Low Body Weight and Weight Loss in the Aged," *Journal of the American Dietetic Association*, v. 90, n. 12, p. 1697, December 1990.

Fischman, Joshua, "Exercise: Getting Your Head in Shape," *Psychology Today*, v. 22, p. 14, January 1988.

"Fixing Wrinkles the Natural Way," *Longevity*, p. 10, March 1993.

"Foods That May Prevent Breast Cancer: Studies Are Investigating Soybeans, Whole Wheat and Green Tea Among Others," *Primary Care and Cancer*, n. 14, pp. 10-11, February 1994.

"For Losing Extra Weight, Try Chromium Picolinate," *Better Nutrition for Today's Living*, v. 56, n. 9, September 1994.

Friedan, Betty, "How to Live Longer, Better, Wiser," *Parade*, p.4, March 20, 1994.

Friedensohn, Aharon, et al., "Malignant Arrhythmias in Relation to Values of Serum Potassium in Patients With Acute Myocardial Infarction," *International Journal of Cardiology*, v. 32, pp. 331-338, 1991.

Friedman, Max, "Food of the Gods," *Vegetarian Times*, n.204, p.58, August 1994.

Fulder, Stephen, "Sniffing Out the Truth About Garlic," *Townsend Letter for Doctors*, p. 1024, November 1992.

G

Gaby, Alan R., M.D., "Commentary," *Nutrition and Healing*, pp. 1, 6, 7, September 1994.

Gaby, Alan, R., M.D.; Wright, Jonathan, V., M.D., *Nutrients and Bone Health*, Wright/Gaby Nutrition Institute, Baltimore, M.D., August 1988.

Gaby, Alan R., *Preventing and Reversing Osteoporosis*, Prima Publishing, Rocklin, Calif., pp. 63-64, 1994.

———., "The Story of Vitamin E," *Nutrition and Healing*, p. 4, October 1994.

———., "Glocosamine Sulfate Effective Treatment for Osteoarthritis," *Townsend Letter for Doctors*, p. 741, July 1993.

Gallagher, Winifred, "Midlife Myths," *Atlantic*, v. 271, May 1993.

Gaziano, J. Michael, "Antioxidant Vitamins and Coronary Artery Disease Risk," *The American Journal of Medicine*, v. 97, September 26, 1994.

Gerber, Paul C., "Alternative Medicine: All Eyes on NIH's Office of Alternative Medicine," *Physician Management*, March 1994.

Gerras, Charles, et al., eds., *The Encyclopedia of Common Diseases*, Rodale Press, Inc. Emmaus, Pa., p. 351, 1976.

Ghersetich, I., et al., *International Journal of Dermatology*, v. 33, n. 2, pp. 119-122, 1994.

Giuliani, A.; Cestaro, B., "Exercise, Free Radical Generation and Vitamins," *European Journal of Cancer Prevention*, v. 6, pp. S55-S67, 1997.

Goldfinger, Stephen E., "Garlic: Good for What Ails You?" *Harvard Health Letter*, v. 16, n. 10, p. 1, August 1991.

"Green Tea Shown to Have Anti-Cancer Effect in Rodents," *Food Chemical News*, v. 36, n. 11, CRC Press, Inc., May 9, 1994.

Grindy, Robert, "More About Magnesium," *Saturday Evening Post*, v. 259, p. 50, July-August 1987.

Gruning, Carl, "Seeing Is Believing! For Lifelong Eye Health, Just Remember Your ABCs and These Minerals," *Health News & Review*, v. 2, n. 3, p. 1, Summer 1992.

Gunby, Phil, "Graying of America Stimulates More Research on Aging-associated Factors," JAMA, *The Journal of the American Medical Association*, v. 272, n. 20, p. 1561, November 23, 1994.

H

Hajdu, David, "Why Not Talk Like a Grown-Up?" *Cosmopolitan*, p. 128, February 1990.

Haney, Daniel, "A Seismic Shift in Heart Care," Associated Press—*The Sacramento Bee*, A1, August 4, 2002.

Hans Kugler, Ph.D., "Tripping the Clock: A Practical Guide to Anti-Aging and Rejuvenation," *Senior Vitality*, April 27, 2000.

Hart, James P.; Cooper, William L., "Vitamin E in the Treatment of Prostate Hypertrophy," Lee Foundation for Nutritional Research, Milwaukee, Wis., Report No. 1, November 1941.

Heinrick, Nat, M.D.; Pecher, Otto, M.D., *Enzymes: A Drug of the Future: Strengthening the Immunological System with Enzyme Therapy*, Dr. Hans Hermann von Wimpffen ecomed, verlagsgesellschaft AG & Co. KG Rudolf-Diesel Str. 3, D-86899 Lansberg/Lech, 1998.

Herbert, Victor, Genell J. Subak-Sharpe, *The Mt. Sinai School of Medicine Complete Book of Nutrition*, St. Martin's Press, New York, 1990.

Herman, Phyllis, "A Natural Way to a Healthy Prostate," *Health News & Review*, v. 3, n. 2, Spring 1993.

Herta, Spencer, M.D., "Inhibitory Effects of Zinc on Magnesium Balance and Magnesium Absorption in Man," *Journal of the American College of Nutrition*, v. 13, n. 5, 1994.

Hertog, M. G. I., et al., "Dietary Antioxidant Flavonoids and Risk of Coronary Heart Disease: the Zutphen Elderly Study," *The Lancet*, v. 342, pp. 1007-1011, 1993.

Higgins, Michael, "Native People Take on Diabetes," *East West*, v. 2,1 n. 4, p. 94, April 1991.

Higgins, Linda C., "Longevity: An Eternal Quest Quickens," *Medical World News*, v. 31, n. 10, p. 22, May 28, 1990.

Hoffman, Matthew & Le Gro, William, *Disease Free*, Rodale Press, pp. 43-45, 1993.

Hoffman, D., *The New Holistic Herbal*, Element Inc., Rockport, Maine, 1991.

Holman, Richard L., "Japanese Longevity Sets Records," *Wall Street Journal*, p. A10, A6, col. 6, July 15, 1994.

Hooper, Judith, "The Hug Factor," *Health*, v. 21, n .10, p. 72, October 1989.

Horrobin, David F., "Review Article: Medical Uses of Essential Fatty Acids (EFAs)," *Veterinary Dermatology*, v. 4, n. 4, pp. 161-166, 1993.

Hudon, Tori, N.D., "A Pilot Study Using Botanical Medicines in the Treatment of Menopausal Symptoms," *Alternative Medicine*, May 1994.

Hunter, Beatrice Trum, "How Well Do We Absorb Nutrients?" *Consumers' Research Magazine*, v. 77, n. 4, p. 17, April 1994.

Hurley, Jayne; Schmidt, Stephen, "Pound Foolish?" *Nutrition Action Healthletter*, v. 18, n. 4, May 1991.

"Hyaluronic Acid," Pentapharm Ltd., Basel, Switzerland.

I

I-San Lin, Robert, "Garlic and Health: Recent Advances in Research," Irvine, Calif., p. 5, 1992.

Imagawa, M., et al., "Coenzyme Q10, Iron and Vitamin B6 in Genetically Confirmed Alzheimer's Disease," *The Lancet*, n. 8820, p. 671, September 1992.

"Intermittant Claudication: Trental vs. Ginkgo Biloba Extract," *American Journal of Natural Medicine*, v. 2, n. 1, p. 12, January/February 1995.

Ishiyama, T., "A Clinical Study of the Effect of Coenzyme Q10 on Congestive Heart Failure," *Jpn Heart J*, v. 17, pp. 32-42, 1976.

J

Jackson, Donald Dale, "From the Lungs to Larynx to Lip, It's Jitter, Shimmer and Blip," *Smithsonian*, p. 78, July 1985.

Jacobson, Stanley, "Attitude: Mind Over Matters," *Modern Maturity*, v. 35, p .36, December-January 1992.

James, Wesley, "Breast Cancer, Have We Lost Our Way?" *World Research Foundation News*, p. 3, First Quarter, 1993.

James, Elizabeth, "Stress: Enemy or Friend?" *Total Health*, v. 13, n. 1, p. 31, February 1991.

Tessler, Gordon S., "The Correct Nutrition to Cope with Stress," *Total Health*, v. 11, n. 3, p. 12, June 1989.

Johnson, Mary Ann and Kays, Sandra E., "Copper: Its Role in Human Nutrition," *Nutrition Today*, v. 25, n. 1, p. 6-15, February 1990.

Judd, A.M., et al., "Zinc Acutely, Selectively and Reversibly Inhibits Pituitary Prolactin Secretion," *Brain Research*, v. 294, 1984.

K

Kadunce, Donald P., M.D., et al., "Cigarette Smoking: Risk Factor For Premature Facial Wrinkling," *Annals of Internal Medicine*, v. 114, n. 10, pp. 840-844, May 15, 1991.

Karvonen, Karen; McCloy, Marjorie; Kort, Michele; O'Rourke, Anne, "Myth Busters: Eight Women Who Prove Aging Doesn't have to Mean Growing Old," *Women's Sports and Fitness*, v. 13 p. 48, October 1991.

Kaufmann, Klaus, *Silica The Forgotten Nutrient*, Alive Books, Barnaby, B.C. Canada, 1990.

Keeton, Kathy, "Mental Muscle," *Omni*, v. 14, p. 40, May 1992.

Kennedy Salaman, Maureen, *Foods that Heal* audiotape, transcript pp.3-6, 8, 11, 14-17, 18-25, 27-29, 33, 1989.

———., *Foods that Heal*, MKS Inc., Menlo Park, Calif., pp. 55-64, 1989.

Kennedy, Bob, "Borage Wildflowers: Best Source of GLA," *Total Health*, v. 13, n. 1, February 1991.

Kidd, Parris M., Ph.D., "An Integrative Lifestyle: Nutritional Strategy For Lowering Osteoporosis Risk," *Townsend Letter for Doctors*, pp. 400-405, May 1992.

Kimble, Melvin A., "Religion: friend or foe of the aging?" *Second Opinion*, v. 15, p. 70, November 1990.

Kintish, Lisa, "Sun Protection: Vitamin A Derivatives, Antioxidants Endorsed at Skin Cancer Foundation Conference," *Soap-Cosmetics-Chemical Specialties*, v. 65, n. 5, p. 17, May 1989.

Koop, C. Everett, "Exploring the Myths and Realities of Aging and Health," *Aging*, p. 4, April-May 1984.

Korpela, Heikki, DVM, M.D., "Hypothesis: Increased Calcium and Decreased Magnesium in Heart Disease and Liver of Pigs Dying Suddenly of Microangiopathy: An Animal Model for the Study of Oxidative Damage," *Journal of the American College of Nutrition*, v. 10, n. 2, pp. 127-131, 1991.

Kugler, Hans J., Ph.D., *Tripping the Clock—A Practical Guide to Anti-Aging and Rejuvenation*, 1992.

————., "A New Approach to Clinical Treatment of Prostate Disorders," *Townsend Letter for Doctors*, April, 1993.

————., et al., *Life Extenders and Memory Boosters*, Health Quest Publications, Reno, Nev., 1993.

L

Laino, Charlene, "Trans-Fatty Acids in Margarine Can Increase MI Risk," *Medical Tribune*, v. 4, February 24, 1994.

Langer, Ellen J., "The Mindset of Health," *Psychology Today*, v. 23, n. 4, p. 48, April 1989.

Langreth, Tobert, "Can We Live to 150?" *Popular Science*, v. 243, p. 77, November 1993.

Lee, John R, M.D., *Natural Progesterone, The Multiple Roles of a Remarkable Hormone*, BLL Publishing, Sebastapol, Calif., May 1995.

————., "Osteoporosis Reversal, The Role of Progesterone," *International Clinical Nutrition Review*, v. 10, n. 3, pp. 384-391, July 1990.

Leguire, Lawrence, et al., "Electro-Oculogram in Vitamin A Deficiency Associated With Cystic Fibrosis," *Ophthalmic Pediatrics*, v. 13, n. 3, pp. 187-189, 1992.

Leibowitz, Sarah, "The Rockefeller University Annual Meeting for the Society of Neuroscience," News Release, Rockefeller University, 1230 York Avenue, New York, N.Y., November 1993.

Levanthal, Lawrence, M.D.; Boyce, Eric G., PharmD; Zurier, Robert B., M.D. "Treatment of Rheumatoid Arthritis with Gammalinolenic Acid," *Annals of Internal Medicine*, v. 119, n. 9, p. 867, November 1993.

Levine, Elyse, "If Longevity Is the Goal, Better Nutrition May Be the Answer," *Environmental Nutrition*, v. 13, n. 2, p. 1, February 1990.

Liebman, Bonnie, "The Best Laid Trans," *Nutrition Action Health Letter*, p. 5, December 1992.

Lippert, Joan, "Wishing Well: A Brave New Science Is Probing the Relationship Between Your Thoughts and Your Health," *Mature Health*, n. 5, p. 24, February 1990.

Lloyd, Tom, Ph.D., et al., "Calcium Supplementation and Bone Mineral Density in Adolescent Girls," *Journal of the American Medical Association*, v. 270, n. 7, August 18, 1993.

Locke, Steven; Cooligan, Daniel, *The Healer Within*, pp. 187-88, E.P. Dutton, New York, 1986.

Londer, Randi, "Anti-Aging Eating; Can the Foods You Eat Keep You Young?" *Health*, v. 18, p. 41, July 1986.

"Longevity Advisor: Menopause Relievers," *Longevity*, February 1993.

Lopez, D.A., M.D., Williams, R.M., M.D., Ph.D., Miehlke, K., M.D., *Enzymes, The Fountain of Life*, The Neville Press, Inc., p. 203, 1999.

Lorenz, H. Peter; Adzick, N. Scott, "Scarless Skin Wound Repair in the Fetus," *The Western Journal of Medicine*, v.159, n. 3, pp. 350-356, September 1993.

Luciano, Lani, "Eight Myths of Retirement," *Money*, v. 19, p. 110, February 1990.

Luskin, Frederic, *Forgive for Good: Seven Steps to Letting Go of Grievances and Hurts*, Stanford Forgiveness Project, 1998.

Lustgarden, Steve, "Flexing Your Mental Muscle," *Vegetarian Times*, n. 183, p. 48, November 1992.

Lux-Neuwirth, Ora; Millar, Thomas J., "Lipid Soluble Antioxidants Preserve Rabbit Corneal Cell Function," *Current Eye Research*, v. 9, n. 2, pp. 103-109, 1990.

M

M.R. Hiller, "Seniors May Benefit from Growth Hormone," The Palo Alto Medical Foundation, 1994.

MacDonald, A.G.; Murphy, E.A.; Capell, H.A.; Bankowska, U.Z.; Ralston, S.H., "Effects of Hormone Replacement Therapy in Rheumatoid Arthritis: A Double Blind Placebo-Controlled Study," *Annals of the Rheumatic Diseases*, pp. 54-57, 1994.

Magnes GD, "Proteolytic Enzymes in Oral Surgery," *Journal of the American Dental Association*, v. 72, pp. 1420-1425, June 1966.

"Magnesium for Acute Myocardial Infarction?" Editor, *The Lancet*, September 14, v. 333, pp. 667-668, September 14, 1991.

Magnesium Can Help With Energy, Depression," *Better Nutrition for Today's Living*, v. 57, n. 2, p. 26, February 1995.

Mandy Behbehani, "Simply Sophia," *San Francisco Examiner*, March 19, 1995.

Mann, George V., "Metabolic Consequences of Dietary Trans Fatty Acids," *Lancet*, v. 343, n. 8908, May 21, 1994.

Mark, Denise Rose, M.D., *Menopause and Andropause (Male Menopause) Hormone Balancing for Women and Men*, South Valley Wellness, 2001.

Martindale, *The Extra Pharmacopoeia, Thirtieth Edition*, Department of Pharmaceutical Sciences, Royal Pharmaceutical Society of Great Britain, The Pharmaceutical Press, 1993.

Marwick, Charles, "Older People Now More Able-bodied Than Before," *JAMA, The Journal of the American Medical Association*, v. 269, p. 2333, May 12, 1993.

Matkovic, V., et al., "Factors that Influence Peak Bone Mass Formation: A Study of Calcium Balance and the Inheritance of Bone Mass in Adolescent Females," *American Journal of Clinical Nutrition*, v. 52, 1990.

McGuire, Rick, "Cancer Prevention Under the Sun," *Total Health*, v. 13, n. 2, April 1991.

"Meat's Risk for Cancer: Just Bologna?...Not When It's Prostate Cancer," *Science News*, v. 145, n. 8, February 19, 1994.

Mervyn, Len, *Minerals and Your Health*, Keats Publishing, pp. 49, 51, 98, 104, 123, 1980.

Merz, Beverly, "Healthy Aging: Why We Get Old," *Harvard Health Letter*, v. 17, n. 12, p. 9, October 1992.

Meyerhoff, Al, "We Must Get Rid of Pesticides in the Food Supply," *USA Today*, p. 51, November 1993.

Miller, Joseph M., M.D.; Opher, Albert W., B.S., "The Increased Proteolytic Activity of Human Blood Serum After the Oral Administration of Bromelain," *Experimental Med. Surg.*, v. 22, n. 4, pp. 277-280, 1964.

Miller, A.B., et al., "Diet in the Etiology of Cancer: A Review," *European Journal of Cancer*, v. 30A, n. 2, 1994.

Millspaugh, Charles F., *American Medicinal Plants*, Dover, New York, 1892/1974.

Mindell, Earl L., "Soy—When Will We Learn?" column "Stay Healthy," *Let's Live*, p. 10, January 1995.

Mitchell, John, "Many Riches to Be Mined from Minerals; Zinc Found Effective Against Many

Ills, Selenium Enhances Immune Response, Silicon May Prevent Alzheimer's Disease," *Health News & Review*, v. 1, n. 2, p. 7, July-August 1991.

Molnar, E. Michael, M.D., *Forever Young*, pp. 79-91, 1985.

Morisco, C., et al., "Effect of Coenzyme Q10 in Patients with Congestive Heart Failure: A Long-Term Multicenter Randomized Study," *Clin Invest*, v. 71, pp. S134-S136, 1993.

Muller, W., et al., "Age-Related Calcium/Magnesium Ratio in the Ligamenta Flava," *Z. Gerontol*, v. 27, pp. 328-329, 1994.

Murray, Frank, "Antioxidants: Health Allies," *Better Nutrition for Today's Living*, v. 54, n. 10, p. 24, October 1992.

———., "Bioflavonoids Add Punch to the Power of Vitamin C," *Better Nutrition*, p. 22, September 1989.

———., "Evening Primrose Oil: Nocturnal Curative Extract," *Better Nutrition for Today's Living*, v. 56, n. 2, p. 34, February 1994.

———., "Keeping an Eye on Good Health," *Today's Living*, v. 20, n. 8, p. 8, August 1989.

———., "Zinc: Healing Mineral," *Better Nutrition for Today's Living*, v.54, n. 9, September 1992.

Murray, Michael, M.D.; Pizzorno, Joseph, N.D., *Encyclopedia of Natural Medicine*, Prima Publishing, Rocklin, Calif., 1991.

Murray, Michael T., *Natural Alternatives to Over-the-Counter and Prescription Drugs*, William Morrow, pp. 74-77, 1994.

N

Neergaard, Lauren, "Breast Cancer Cases Top Malpractice Suits," *Associated Press*, June 3, 1995.

Nelson, Rebecca, "Age is an Attitude," *Woman's Day*, v. 56, p. 68, Febuary 2, 1993.

"New Evidence for Aluminium/Alzheimer's Link," *SCRIP World Pharmaceutical News*, n. 1918, p. 22, April 29, 1994.

Newbold, H. L, *Mega-Nutrients*, p. 347, The Body Press, Los Angeles, 1987.

Nielsen, F. H., "Boron, an Overlooked Element of Potential Nutrition Importance," *Nutrition Today*, pp. 4-7, January/February 1988.

Null, Gary, *The Complete Guide to Health and Nutrition*, Dell Publishing Inc., New York, 1984.

O

Offenbacher, E. G., et al., "Promotion of Chromium Absorption by Ascorbic Acid," *Trace Elements and Electrolytes*, v. 11, n. 4, 1994.

Olshansky, S. Jay; Carnes, Bruce A.; Cassel, Christine, "In Search of Methuselah: Estimating the Upper Limits to Human Longevity," *Science*, v. 250, n. 4981, p. 634, November 2, 1990.

Orlov, Michael, M.D., et al., "A Review of Magnesium, Acute Myocardial Infarction Arrhythmia," *The Journal of the American College of Nutrition*, v. 13, n. 2, pp. 127-132, 1994.

P

Panayi, G. S. "Phototherapy—T Cell Vaccination by Any Other Name?" *Clin. Exp. Immunol*, pp. 363-365, 1994.

Parachin, Victor M., "Facts of Life: A Dozen Ways to Live Longer and Better," *American Fitness*, v. 12, n. 1, p. 42, January-February 1994.

Passwater, Richard A., "Neglected Trace Mineral May Increase Lifespan," *Health News & Review*, v. 3, n. 2, Spring 1993.

Pearson, Durk; Shaw, Sandy, "Save Our Skin," *LifeNet News*, v. 3, n. 7, p. 10, July 1992.

Peehl, Donna M., et al., "Vitamin A Regulates Proliferation and Differentiation of Human Prostatic Epithelial Cells," *The Prostate*, v. 23, 1993.

———., et al., "Vitamin D and Prostate Cancer," *Journal of Endocrinology Investigation*, v. 17, 1994.

Pennington, Jean A. T., Ph.D., RD; Young, Barbara E., "Total Diet Study of Nutritional Elements, 1982-1989," *Journal of The American Dietetic Association*, v. 91, n. 2, pp. 179-183, February 1991.

Perricone, N., et al., "Alpha Lipoic Acid (ALA) Protects Proteins Against the Hydroxyl Free Radical-Induced Alterations: Rationale for Its Geriatric Topical Application," *Arch Gerontol Geriatr*, v. 29, pp. 45-56, 1999.

"Personality—The Key to Living Longer," *Executive Health's Good Health Report*, v. 30, n. 4, p. 8, January 1994.

"Pharmacologic Doses of Vitamin E Improve Insulin Action in Healthy Subjects and Non-Insulin-Dependent Diabetic Patients," *American Journal of Clinical Nutrition*, May 1993.

"Population Health Looking Upstream," *The Lancet*, v. 343, n. 8895, p. 429, February 19, 1994.

"Postmenopausal Hormone Therapy," *HealthFacts*, Center for Medical Consumers, New York, N.Y., May 1991.

Prevention Magazine, The Encyclopedia of Common Diseases, pp. 81, 83, 85, 89, 92, 100-103, April 1984.

Prielipp, Richard C., M.D., et al., "Magnesium Antagonizes the Action of Lyso-phosphatidylcholine (LPC) in Myocardial Cells: A Possible Mechanism For Its Antiarrhythmic Effects," *Anesth Analg*, v. 80, pp. 1083-1087, 1995.

R

Rae, Stephen, "Wrapping the Human Package," p. 91, *Mademoiselle*, June-July 1991.

Rai, G., et al., "Double-Blind, Placebo-Controlled Study of Acetyl-L-Carnitine in Patients with Alzheimer's Dementia," *Current Medical Resident Opinion*, v. 11, p. 638, 1990.

Raloff, J., "Margarine Is Anything but a Marginal Fat," *Science News*, v. 145, p. 325, May 21, 1994.

Rattenbury, Jeanne, "Mind-body Mania," *Vegetarian Times*, n. 195, p. 74, November 1993.

"Recent Research Supports the Cardiovascular and Cancer Protective Benefits of Garlic," press release, May 27, 1994.

"Research Offers Evidence of Vitamin E Cardiac Benefit," *Medical Tribune*, p. 8, November 21, 1994.

"Research Shows Garlic Inhibits Breast Cancer," *Daily Standard*, Celina, Ohio, February 25, 1994.

Riggs, Lawrence B., M.D. and Melton, Joseph L., III, M.D., "The Prevention and Treatment of Osteoporosis," *New England Journal of Medicine*, v. 327, n. 9, August 27, 1992.

Robins, Cynthia, "Oh, to Be Sophia," *San Francisco Examiner*, April 4, 1995.

Rodale, J.I. *Complete Book of Minerals for Health*, Rodale Press, pp. 735, 1975.

Rodgers, George M., "Novel Antithrombotic Therapy," *The Western Journal of Medicine*, v. 159, n. 6, p. 670, December 1993.

Rose, Richard; Dode, Ann M., "Ocular Ascorbate Transport Metabolism," *Comp. Biochem. Physiol.*, v. 108, n. 2, pp. 273-285, 1991.

Ross, Julia, M.A., *The Diet Cure*, Penguin Books, 1999.

Rubin, Rita, "Placebos' Healing Power: Pills That Shouldn't Work Often Do Anyway," *U.S. News & World Report*, v. 115, n. 20, p. 78, November 22, 1993.

Russell, Robert M., "Nutrition," *JAMA, The Journal of the American Medical Association*, June 1, 1994.

S

Sahley, Bille J.; Birkner, Kathy, "Stress and Menopause," *Total Health*, v. 10, n. 5, p. 54, October 1988.

Saltman, P., "The Role of Minerals and Osteoporosis," *Journal of the American College of Nutrition*,

v. 11, n. 5, p. 599, October 1992.

Schneider, Edward, "Biological Theories of Aging," *Generations*, v. 16, n. 4, p. 7, Fall-Winter, 1992.

Scott-Samuel, Alex, "Health Promotion Research: Towards a New Social Epidemiology," *British Medical Journal*, v. 305, n. 6853, p. 593, September 5, 1992.

Seelig, Mildred S., M.D., M.P.H., "Magnesium, Antioxidants and Myocardial Infarction," *American Journal of Clinical Nutrition*, v. 13, n. 2, pp. 116-117, 1994.

———., et al., "Consequences of Magnesium Deficiency on Enhancement of Stress Reaction; Preventive and Therapeutic Implications (A Review)," *Journal of the American College of Nutrition*, v. 13, n. 5, pp. 429-446, 1994.

Selhub, Jacob and Paul F. Jacques, et. al., "Association Between Plasma Homocysteine Concentrations and Extracranial Carotid Artery Stenosis," *New England Journal of Medicine*, v. 332, n. 5, pp. 286-291, February 2, 1995.

Selkoe, Dennis J., "Aging Brain, Aging Mind," *Scientific American*, v. 267 p. 134, September 1992.

Seyle, Hans, *Calciphylaxis*, University of Chicago Press, Chicago, Illinois, 1962.

Shreeve, Caroline M., *The Alternative Dictionary of Symptoms and Cures*, Century Paperbacks, pp. 312, 315, 317, August 1999.

Skow, John, "It's Coming Back to Me Now! At 42, George Foreman is duking it out..." *Time*, v. 137, p. 78, April 22, 1991.

Smith, C. J. "Non-Hormonal Control of VasoMotor Flushing in Menopausal Patients," *Chicago Medicine*, March 7, 1964.

Snowdon, David, *Aging With Grace: What the Nun Study Teaches Us About Leading Longer, Healthier, and More Meaningful Lives*, Bantam Doubleday Dell Publications, April 30, 2002.

Sobel, Dava, "The 120-year Man: By Undereating, Roy Walford Plans to Beat the Longevity Odds," *American Health: Fitness of Body and Mind*, v. 10, n. 7, p. 18, September 1991.

Stampfer, Meir J.; Rene M. Malinow, "Can Lowering Homocysteine Levels Reduce Cardiovascular Risk?" *New England Journal of Medicine*, v. 332, n. 5, pp. 28-29, February 2, 1995.

Stephens, N.G., et al., "Randomized Controlled Trial of Vitamin E in Patients with Coronary Disease: Cambridge Heart Antioxidant Study (CHAOS), *The Lancet*, v. 347, pp. 781-786, March 23, 1996.

Straus, Hal, "The Lazarus File: When the 'Spontaneous' Cure Comes from Within," *American Health: Fitness of Body and Mind*, v. 8, n. 4, p. 67, May 1989.

Subak-Sharpe, Genell, J.; Bogdonoff, Morton, D., *Home Health Handbook*, BV/IMP, Inc, pp. 37, 45, MCMLXXXXIX.

Superko, H. Robert, "Amino Acid Defect Causes 20 Percent of Atherosclerosis in CHD," *Family Practice News*, p.7, October 15, 1994.

T

"Tapping Human Potential," *Second Opinion*, v. 14, p. 56, July 1990.

Tassman, Gustav, D.D.S., et al., "Evaluation of a Plant Proteolytic Enzyme For the Control of Inflammation and Pain," *Journal of Dental Disease*, v. 19, pp. 73-77, 1964.

Taylor, Deborah Semour, "Hypoglycemia Responds to Natural Treatment," *Better Nutrition*, v. 51, n. 10, p. 13, October 1989.

Teresi, Dick, "Wanted: Forty More Years," *Health*, v. 21, n. 10, p. 58, October 1989.

Terry, Cass, M.D., Ph.D., Pharm.D., Medical College of Wisconsin, Milwaukee; Chein, Edmund, M.D., Palm Springs Life Extension Institute, Palm Springs, CA, *Human Growth Hormone Replacement Therapy in Aging Adults*, a paper presented at the Fourth Annual

Convention of the American Academy of Anti-Aging Medicine, Alexis Park Resort, Las Vegas, Nev., December 14-16, 1996.

"The Mysteries of Melatonin," *Harvard Health Letter*, June 1993.

Thogersen, Anna M., et al., "Effects of Intravenous Magnesium Sulfate in Suspected Acute Myocardial Infarction on Acute Arrhythmias and Long-Term Outcome," *International Journal of Cardiology*, v. 49, pp. 143-151, 1995.

Thomas, Patricia, "Vitamin C Eyed for Topical Use as Skin Preserver; the Compound Appears to ward off Sun Damage, and the Developer Thinks It May Promote Collagen Synthesis," *Medical World News*, v. 32, n. 3, p. 12, March 1991.

Thomson, Bill, "In Search of Longevity," *East West*, v. 19, n .12, p. 42, December 1989.

Thorne Research, "Acetyl-L-Carnitine," Thorne Research Abstracts, February 17, 1995.

Tisserand, Robert, article on tea tree oil, *The International Journal of Aromatherapy*, February 1988.

Todd, Susan, et al., "An Investigation of the Relationship Between Antioxidant Vitamin Intake and Coronary Heart Disease in Men and Women Using Logistic Regression Analysis," *Journal of Clinical Epidemiology*, v. 48, n. 2, pp. 307-316, 1995.

Tomita, A., "Postmenopausal Osteoporosis Calcium Kinetic Study with Vitamin K in Osteoporosis," *Clin Endocrinol Metab*, v. 60, pp. 1268-1269, 1985.

"Topical Bioactive Materials," *Cosmetics and Toiletries*, September 1994.

Toufexis, Anastasia, "Older — But Coming on Strong; Aging No Longer Has to Mean Sickness, Senility and Sexlessness," *Time*, v. 131, p. 76, February 22, 1988.

Touyz, R. M., "Magnesium Supplementation as an Adjuvant to Synthetic Calcium Channel Antagonism in the Treatment of Hypertension," *Medical Hypothesis*, v. 36, pp. 140-141, 1991.

Townley, Wyatt. "Exercise Update," *Cosmopolitan*, pp. 162-165, 215, August 1993.

Treating Prostate Problems, a booklet, Krames Communications, San Bruno, Calif., 1991.

Tufts University Diet & Nutrition Letter, v. 10, n. 11, p. 3, January 1993.

"Twenty Super Foods Wipe Out Wrinkles," *The Examiner*, p. 19, June 11, 1991.

U

"Urinary Selenium Concentrations," *Clinical Chemistry*, v. 39, n. 10, 1993.

V

Velioglu Y. S., et al., "Antioxidant Activity and Total Phenolics in Selected Fruits, Vegetables, and Grain Products," *Journal of Agricultural and Food Chemistry*, v. 46, pp. 4113-4117, 1998.

Vikhanski, L. E., "Magnesium May Slow Bone Loss," *Medical Tribune*, July 22, 1993.

Viorst, Judith, "Getting Older, Growing Younger," *Saturday Evening Post*, v. 257, p. 62 January-February 1985.

————., "Fortysomething Is a Wonderful Age!" *Redbook*, v. 173 p. 42, June 1989.

"Vitamin B12 and Alzheimer's Disease," *The Nutrition Report*, v. 75, p. 12, October 1994.

Voelker, Rebecca, "Recommendations for antioxidants: how much evidence is enough?" *JAMA, The Journal of the American Medical Association*, v. 271, n. 15, p. 1148, April 20, 1994.

Vukovic, Laurel, "Aging Gracefully: Natural Approaches to Maintain Your Vitality," *Natural Health*, v. 23, n. 4, p. 86, July-August 1993.

W

Wade, Carlson, *Inner Cleansing*, Prentice Hall Trade, pp. 22-23, September 1992.

Walker, Morton. "Non-Toxic Symptomatic Arthritis Relief Using Sea Cucumber," *Townsend*

Letter for Doctors, p. 650, October 1990.

Wang, Hong, et al., "Total Antioxidant Capacity of Fruits," *Journal of Agricultural and Food Chemistry*, v. 44, pp. 701-705, 1996.

Werbach, Melvyn R., *Nutritional Influences on Illness*, Keats Publishing, New Canaan, Conn., 1988.

Whitaker, Julian, "Preventing Breast Cancer," *Health and Healing*, January 1994.

White, Kristin, "How the Mind Ages," *Psychology Today*, v. 26, p. 38, November-December 1993.

Wilcox, Gisela, et al., "Oestrogenic Effects of Plant Foods in Postmenopausal Women," *British Medical Journal*, v. 301, n. 6757, October 20, 1990.

Willett, Walter C., et al., "Intake of Trans Fatty Acids and Risk of Coronary Heart Disease Among Women," *The Lancet*, v. 341, pp. 581-585, March 6, 1993.

Woods, Kent L.; Fletcher, Susan; Roffe, Christine; Haider, Yasser, "Intravenous Magnesium Sulphate in Suspected Acute Myocardial Infarction: Results of the Second Leicester Intravenous Magnesium Intervention Trial," *The Lancet*, v. 339, n. 8809, p. 1553, June 27, 1992.

Wright, Jonathan, "Congestive Heart Failure," *Nutrition & Healing*, v. 1, n. 5, December 1994.

Wright, Jonathan, M.D., *Dr. Wright's Book of Nutritional Therapy*, Rodale Press, Emmaus, Pa., 1979.

X

Xia, Yiming, et al., "Keshan's Disease and Selenium Status of Populations in China," *Selenium in Biology and Human Health*, Chapter 10, pp. 183-196, 1994.

Y

Yamasaki, Takeshi, et al., "Garlic Compounds Protect Vascular Endothelial Cells from Hydrogen Peroxide-Induced Oxidant Injury," *Phytotherapy Research*, v. 8, pp.4 08-412, 1994.

Yiamouyiannis, John, *Fluoride: The Aging Factor*, Health Action Press, Delaware, Ohio, p. 4, 1983.

Yokel, Robert A., "Aluminum Exposure Produces Learning and Memory Deficits: A Model of Alzheimer's Disease," *Toxin-Induced Models of Neurologic Disorders*, Woodruff, Michael L. and Nonneman, Arthury, Plenum Press, chpt. 11, p. 301, 1994.

Z

Zeavin, Edna, "Foods that Influence Behavior," *Bestways*, p. 11, September 1985.

Zucker, Martin. "Ancient Indian Medical Herb Proving Itself a Winner for Modern-Day "Arthritis Sufferers," *Townsend Letter for Doctors*, p. 874, August/September 1993.

INDEX

T

X

Y

Z

W

A special thanks goes to Cher Mullen—
For bringing this creation through the channel of birth to life!

MAUREEN KENNEDY SALAMAN